I0442051

2016

THE AUSTRALIAN

SUGAR

FREE

SHOPPER'S GUIDE

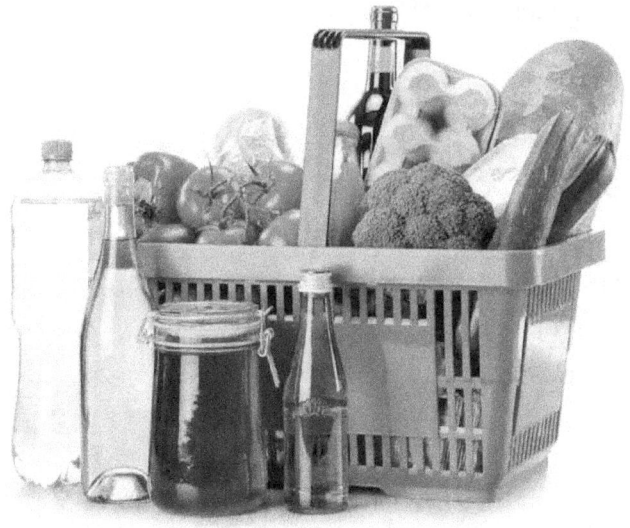

DAVID GILLESPIE

Contents

Break the Sugar Habit

Governments spend a fortune on programs aimed at making us lose weight. They tell us to eat less fatty food and exercise more. Meanwhile we fork over ever-increasing amounts on gym memberships, packaged meals, books, magazines and the advice of experts. Despite decades of this we are now fatter than at any other time in history.

Increasingly the signs are that sugar, or more specifically, fructose (the sugar in fruit, and one half of table sugar), is the culprit behind the obesity crisis.

The Important Sugars

There are only three important simple sugars: glucose, fructose and galactose. All of the other sugars you are likely to encounter in daily life are simply combinations of these three.

Glucose is by far the most plentiful of the simple sugars. Pretty much every food (except meat) contains significant quantities of glucose. Even meat (protein) is eventually converted to glucose by our digestive system. It's a pretty important sugar to humans, as it is our primary fuel – no glucose means no us.

Galactose is present in our environment in only very small quantities and is found mainly in dairy products in the form of lactose (where it is joined to a glucose molecule).

Fructose is also relatively rare in nature. It is found primarily in ripe fruits, which is why it is sometimes call fruit sugar. It is usually found together with glucose and it is what makes food taste sweet. As well as fruit, it's naturally present in honey (40%), Maple Syrup (35%) and Agave Syrup (90%).

Sucrose is what we think of when someone says table sugar. It's one half glucose and one half fructose. Brown sugar, caster sugar, raw sugar and Low GI sugar are all just sucrose.

A very new and deadly addition to our diet

Two hundred years ago, the only way you could eat a significant amount of fructose was to be the king of England or to come into the small fortune required to buy sugar or honey. But now every person in Australia is eating around 50 kilograms of sugar (25 kilograms of fructose) a year.

Soft-drink and fruit juice consumption alone has increased by 30 percent in just the last two decades and two thirds of the adult population is now overweight or obese. Today our collective weight problem continues to accelerate in direct proportion to our consumption of sugar.

A slew of recent research makes it clear that as a species we are ill-equipped to deal with the relatively large amounts of sugar (and therefore fructose) we now consume.

The research shows we have one primary appetite-control centre in our brain called the hypothalamus. It reacts to four major appetite hormones. Three of these hormones tell us when we have had enough to eat and one of them temporarily inhibits the effect of the other three and tells us that we need to eat.

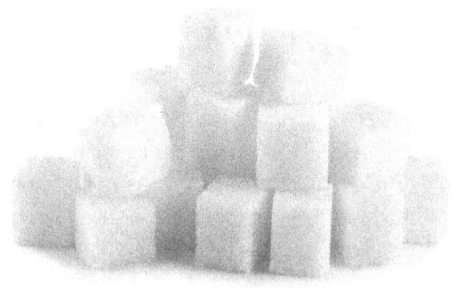

Fructose, uniquely among the food we eat, will not stimulate the release of any of the 'enough to eat' hormones. So we can eat it (and any food containing it) without feeling full. Worse still, fructose is not used for energy by our bodies. Instead all of the fructose is directly converted to fat by our livers. This means that by the time we finish our glass of apple juice (or cola or chocolate bar) the first mouthful will already be circulating in our bloodstream as fat.

Just to put the icing on the cake, recent research has now confirmed what most chocolate lovers have always suspected – sugar is as addictive as cocaine.

How to tell if you're addicted to sugar

Do you struggle to walk past a sugary treat without taking 'just one'?

Do you have routines around sugar consumption – for example, always having pudding or needing a piece of chocolate to relax in front of the TV or treating yourself to a sweet drink or chocolate after a session at the gym?

Are there are times when you feel as if you cannot go on without a sugar hit?

If you are forced to go without sugar for 24 hours, do you develop headaches and mood swings?

Obesity is just symptom of a litany of diseases caused by our fructose addiction. Some diseases are directly related to increased body weight, such as osteoarthritis, fractures, hernia and sleep apnoea. Some are related to the way in which fructose messes with our hormones, such as acne and polycystic ovary syndrome. Others are caused by the fructose induced flood of blood-borne fatty acids, notably cardiovascular diseases, fatty liver disease and type II diabetes. And recent research is also suggesting our overindulgence in fructose is directly linked to a variety of cancers, chronic kidney disease, erectile dysfunction and Alzheimer's disease.

Avoiding Fructose

The addictive ingredient in sugar is the fructose. And because it is addictive, food manufacturers have included it in just about everything.

Getting Fructose Out of Your Diet

Breaking a sugar addiction means that before you even start you've got to pick your way through a minefield of fructose filled foods. But in every category of foods there are some which are much lower in fructose than others. This Guide is all about helping you find those low fructose foods.

We know how difficult it is to stop smoking. Imagine how hard it would be if everything we ate or drank contained nicotine. Because much of our food is laced with fructose, breaking a sugar habit is far harder than giving up smoking. But if you use this guide to help with the shopping, you will have avoided most dietary fructose.

The rules for including a food are pretty simple:

1. **Drinks must have no fructose per 100ml.**

2. **Foods must have less than 1.5g of fructose per 100g (less than 3g per 100g of 'Sugars' on the label)**

The reason for the harsh limit on drinks is that we usually drink much more than 100ml at a time. A can of soft drink is 375 ml, a bottle is 600 ml and some fast food outlets serve soft drink in 1 litre sizes. Foods on the other hand are often served at or around the hundred gram mark (except yoghurts and ice-creams which are usually 200 g).

The label on the food is the primary source for information about fructose content. "Sugars" on the label are assumed to be sucrose (glucose + fructose) unless the ingredients list indicates otherwise. For example, dairy foods will often contain considerable quantities of lactose (galactose + glucose) which will appear under the heading 'Sugars'. Those foods have the probable lactose content deducted from the sugar's total before fructose content is calculated.

If a food is not in this list then it is either too high in fructose or I am not aware of it (please send me an email david@davidgillespie.org) to let me know about any missing foods.

Only processed foods are included in the list. If you plan to eat whole food only, then you don't need to know the sugar content, just keep fruit to a minimum (less than 2 pieces per day or 1 for a child). Juice or dried versions are not acceptable substitutes for whole fruit or vegetables.

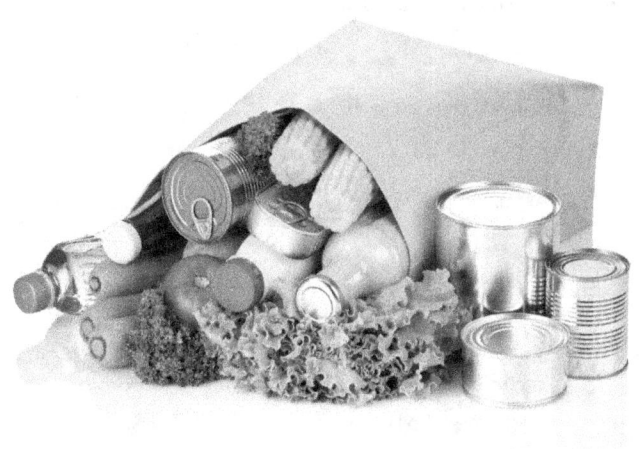

Sugar Substitutes

I'm not a big fan of the term artificial sweetener. It implies that other sweeteners (such as sugar, or fruit juice or high fructose corn syrup) are in some way natural, with all the goodness we have been conditioned to imply into that term. And there is nothing natural about extracting sugar from sugar cane. Substitute sweetener strikes me as a more appropriate description. They are substitutes for sugar, intended to do the job of sugar. In reality sugar itself is a substitute sweetener (for honey) but let's not get all technical. They are all created by using various levels of technology (from manmade beehives to industrial chemical plants) with the sole purpose of adding sweet taste to foods which are not otherwise sweet.

There are three categories of substitute sweetener; those that are absolutely safe to consume; and those that may be safe in limited doses and those which are not safe under any circumstances (usually because they are metabolized to fructose anyway).

Substitute Sweeteners commonly used in Australia

Good	Your call	Bad	
Corn Syrup	Acesulphame potassium (#950)	Agave Syrup	Mannitol (#421)
Dextrose	Alitame (#956)	Fructose	Maple Syrup
Glucose	Aspartame (#951)	Fruit Juice Extract	Molasses
Glucose Syrup	Aspartame-acesuphame (#962)	Golden Syrup	Polydextrose
Lactose	Cyclamates (#952)	High Fructose Corn Syrup	Resistant (malto) dextrin
Maltose	Erythritol (#968)	Honey	Sorbitol (#420)
Maltodextrin	Neotame (#961)	Inulin	Sucrose
Maltodextrose	Saccharin (#954)	Isomalt (#953)	Wheat dextrin
Rice Malt Syrup	Stevia (#960)	Lactitol (#966)	
	Sucralose (#955)	Litesse	
	Xylitol (#967)	Maltitol (#965)	

Seed Oils

The lists that follow are based entirely on sugar content alone. I have also written about the dangers of some types of vegetable oil (seed oils) in my books *Big Fat Lies*, *Toxic Oil* and *Eat Real Food*. Some of the products in the lists below will contain seed oils, but as food manufacturers are not required to label the exact fats that they are using in a product, I have not included information about the fats in these lists. We can however have an educated guess and if you are concerned about the seed oil content of any product, I encourage you to use my fat ready reckoner chart available at www.howmuchsugar.com.

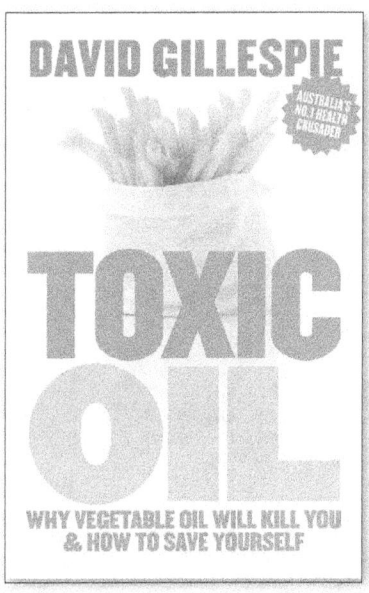

The Lists

Muesli Bars

No qualifying products.

The Atkins Advantage brand of bars are very low in sugar but use artificial sweeteners which are metabolized to fructose (the one's on the 'your call' list on previous page).

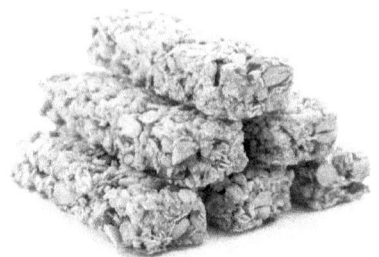

Drinks

The only qualifying products are unsweetened tea or coffee, diet soft drinks, water and milk (both whole and low fat).

The only branded soft drink which qualifies as low fructose is Lucozade Original. It is sweetened with glucose (only) and therefore contains no fructose.

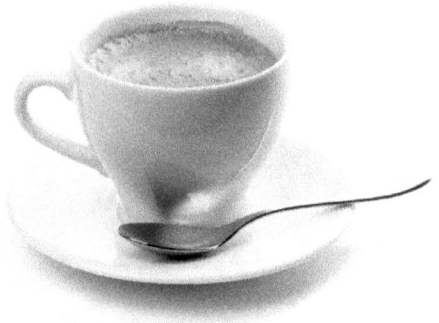

Confectionery

All of the following products have been sweetened with glucose rather than sugar (sucrose).

Brand	Label
Wonka (Nestle)	Runts
	Bottle Caps
	Everlasting Gobstopper
	Chewy Gobstopper
	Gobstopper Snowballs
Frusano	Filita Organic Whole Milk Chocolate
	Organic-Filita Amaranth
	Organic Rice-Crispies
	Filita Organic Dark Chocolate
	Organic Fili-Bears (Gummi Bears)
	Organic Blackberry Candies
	Organic Peppermint Candies
	Ricemalt peppermint hard candy
	Ricemalt lemon hard candy
	Ricemalt orange hard candy
	Dextrose Lolly
Funtastic	Groovy Candy Rolls

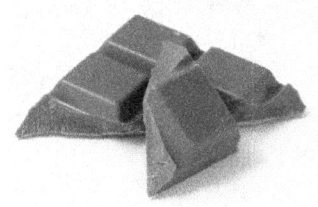

Table Sauces

Brand	Label	% Sugar
	MAYONNAISE*	
S&W	Garlic Traditional Aioli	0.2 %
Country Cuisine	Roasted Garlic Aioli	0.4 %
S&W	Organic Whole Egg Mayonnaise	0.9 %
Best Foods	Real Mayonnaise	1.0 %
Cucina Antica	Maionese della casa	1.0 %
Norganic	Golden Soya Mayonnaise	1.0 %
S&W	Real Whole Egg Mayonnaise	1.0 %
Paul Newman's Own	Classic Whole Egg Aioli	1.1 %
Paul Newman's Own	Whole Egg Aioli	1.1 %
Paul Newman's Own	Whole Egg Mayonnaise	1.1 %
Thomy	Delikatess Mayonnaise	1.1 %
Colway	Real Mayonnaise	1.2 %
Woolworths Select	Whole Egg Mayonnaise	1.2 %
Hellmann's	Real Mayonnaise	1.3 %
Zoosh	Free Range Egg Garlic Aioli	1.7 %
Zoosh	Free Range Egg Peri Mayo	1.8 %
Blessed & Lucky	Free Range Egg Garlicky Aioli	1.9 %
Zoosh	Free Range Egg Mayonnaise	1.9 %
Blessed & Lucky	Free Range Egg Mayonnaise	2.0 %
Zoosh	Free Range Egg Light Mayonnaise	2.1 %
Hellmann's	Light Mayonnaise	2.2 %
Praise	Real Whole Egg Mayonnaise	2.2 %
S&W	Real Whole Egg Light Mayonnaise	2.5 %
Colway	Creamy Aioli	2.6 %

Brand	Label	% Sugar
S&W	Light Real Mayonnaise	2.6 %
Heinz	Seriously Good Garlic Aioli Mayonnaise	3.0 %
Heinz	Seriously Good Whole Egg Mayonnaise	3.0 %
Woolworths Macro Organic	Whole Egg Mayonnaise	3.0 %
Global Organics	Strong Dijon Mustard	0.0 %
	MUSTARD	
Global Organics	Wholegrain Mustard	0.0 %
Maille	Dijon Originale Mustard	0.0 %
Temeraire	Wholegrain Mustard	0.0 %
Masterfoods	Hot English Mustard	0.1 %
Masterfoods	Australian Mustard	0.3 %
Tania	Dijon Mustard	0.8 %
The Regimental Condiment Company	Mustang Dijon Mustard	1.1 %
Masterfoods	Mild English Mustard	1.2 %
Woolworths Macro Organic	Wholegrain Mustard	1.4 %
Woolworths Select	Dijon Mustard	1.4 %
Mrs Bridges	Balsamic Mustard	1.5 %
Tania	Dijon Seeded Mustard	1.5 %
Woolworths Gold	Burgundy Mustard	1.6 %
Woolworths Gold	Wholegrain Mustard	1.8 %
Woolworths Macro Organic	Dijon Mustard	1.9 %
Spiral Foods	French Organic Wholegrain Mustard	2.0 %
Maille	Wholegrain Squeezy Mustard	2.1 %
Masterfoods	French Mustard	2.2 %

Brand	Label	% Sugar
Woolworths Select	Wholegrain Mustard	2.3 %
Maille	Dijon Originale Squeezy Mustard	2.6 %
Spiral Foods	French Organic Dijon Mustard	2.6 %
Moutarde	Extra Strong Dijon Mustard	2.7 %
Temeraire	Dijon Mustard	2.7 %
Moutarde	Wholegrain Mustard	2.8 %
HOT SAUCES		
Cholula	Original Hot Sauce	0.0 %
Ranchero	Salsa Caliente	0.0 %
Ranchero	Salsa De Chipotle	0.0 %
Frank's	RedHot Xtra Hot Cayenne Pepper Sauce	0.5 %
La Costena	Red Jalapeno Hot Sauce	0.5 %
Tapatio	Salsa Picante Hot Sauce	0.7 %
McIlhenney	Tobasco Sauce	1.1 %
Woolworths Select	Portuguese Style Peri Peri Sauce	1.2 %
Byron Bay Chilli Co.	Red Cayenne Chilli Sauce	1.6 %
Frank's	RedHot Original Cayenne Pepper Sauce	1.7 %
Fountain	Good Choice Sweet Chilli Sauce	2.4 %
Byron Bay Chilli Co.	Green Jalapeno Chilli Sauce	2.7 %
ASIAN		
Abundant Earth	Tamari Reduced Salt Soy Sauce	0.0 %
Ayam	Fish Sauce	0.0 %
Pandaroo	Fish Sauce	0.0 %
Spiral Foods	Shoyu Organic Soy Sauce	0.5 %
Spiral Foods	Shoyu Soy Sauce	0.5 %
Spiral Foods	Tamari Organic Soy Sauce	0.5 %
Spiral Foods	Tamari Salt Reduced Soy Sauce	0.5 %

Brand	Label	% Sugar
Spiral Foods	Tamari Soy Sauce	0.5 %
Yeo's	Light Soya Sauce	0.5 %
Thai Gourmet	Fish Sauce	1.1 %
Kikkoman	Soy Sauce	1.3 %
Squid Brand	Fish Sauce	1.3 %
Asia Specialties	Japanese Style Soy Sauce	1.8 %
Kikkoman	Gluten Free Soy Sauce	1.9 %
Kikkoman	Organic Soy Sauce	2.3 %
Coles	Soy Sauce	2.6 %
Pureharvest	Organic Tamari Traditional Soy Sauce	2.6 %
Fountain	Soy & Garlic Sauce	2.9 %
Fountain	Soy Sauce	2.9 %
Pearl River Bridge	Superior Light Soy Sauce	3.0 %
	DRESSINGS*	
Walden Farms	Caesar Salad Dressing	0.5 %
Walden Farms	Honey Dijon Salad Dressing	0.5 %
Walden Farms	Italian Salad Dressing	0.5 %
Cardini's	Original Caesar Dressing	1.0 %
Paul Newman's Own	Creamy Caesar Dressing	1.8 %
Ozganics	Creamy Caesar Dressing	2.2 %
Paul Newman's Own	Classic Dressing	2.9 %

* All of the Mayonnaises and Dressings are made using seed oils and should be avoided or minimized if you are concerned about consuming them.

Cook In Sauces

Brand	Label	% Sugar
	ASIAN	
Celebrate Health	Chinese Beef Stirfry	0.5 %
Celebrate Health	Teriyaki Chicken Stirfry	0.6 %
Maggi	Original Seasoning	2.6 %
Sharwood's	Chinese Curry Cooking Sauce	2.9 %
Yeo's	Malaysian Curry Sauce	1.0 %
	INDIAN	
Sharwood's	Extra Onions Tikka Masala	1.1 %
Passage Foods	Sri Lankan Chicken Curry Simmer Sauce	1.5 %
Sharwood's	Lime Pickle Cooking Sauce	1.6 %
The Spice Tailor	Spiced Spinach Curry	1.9 %
Celebrate Health	Indian Butter Chicken	2.1 %
Margaret Rowland	Indian Vindaloo Simmer Sauce	2.1 %
Naked Curry	Korma Curry Base	2.3 %
Passage Foods	Street Kitchen Coconut Chicken Chettinad	2.4 %
Margaret Rowland	Indian Biriyani Simmer Sauce	2.5 %
Naked Curry	Rogan Josh Curry Base	2.6 %
Sharwood's	Vindaloo Cooking Sauce	2.6 %
The Spice Tailor	Mangalore Herb Curry	2.9 %
Ozganics	Indian Tikka Masala Curry Sauce	3.0 %
The Spice Tailor	Keralan Coconut Curry	3.0 %
	ITALIAN	
Leggo's	Providore Parmesan, Emmental, Mascarpone and Roquefort Sauce	0.5 %

Brand	Label	% Sugar
Five Brothers	Dante's Creamy Bacon with Parmesan Cheese Pasta Bake	1.5 %
ME'N'U	Chunky Bolognese Sauce	1.5 %
Five Brothers	Christophe's White Lasagne Sauce	1.6 %
Five Brothers	Christophe's Provvista Sugo Classica	1.8 %
Global Organics	Tomato Puree Passata	1.8 %
Leggo's	Tomato, Ricotta & Spinach Pasta Bake	1.8 %
Leggo's	Alfredo Pasta Sauce	1.9 %
Biofood Organic	Natural Italian Sauce	2.0 %
Leggo's	Carbonara Pasta Sauce	2.1 %
Leggo's	Tomato, Olive & Chilli Stir Through Sauce	2.1 %
Leggo's	Tuna Bake Spinach & Garlic Pasta Bake	2.1 %
Raguletto	Classic Tomato Bolognese Pasta Sauce	2.1 %
Coles	Creamy Carbonara Fresh Pasta Sauce	2.2 %
Coles	Tomato, Onion & Garlic Fresh Pasta Sauce	2.4 %
Leggo's	Bechamel Lasagne Sauce	2.5 %
Leggo's	Italian Chicken Scallopini Simmer Sauce	2.5 %
Casa Barelli	Creamy Tuna Pasta Bake	2.6 %
Leggo's	Tomato & Garlic with Red Wine Stir Through Sauce	2.6 %
Coles	Creamy Tomato & Basil Pasta Bake	2.7 %
Leggo's	Creamy Sundried Tomato & Garlic Pasta Bake	2.7 %
Leggo's	Creamy Tomato & Mozzarella Pasta Bake	2.7 %

Brand	Label	% Sugar
Leggo's	Providore Italian Tomatoes with Whole Cherry Tomatos & Chilli	2.7 %
Leggo's	Ricotta, Spinach & Pecorino Cheese Stir Through Sauce	2.7 %
Leggo's	Bolognese with Bacon Pasta Sauce	2.9 %
Leggo's	Bolognese with Mushroom Pasta Sauce	2.9 %
Passage Foods	Creamy Broccoli, Spinach & Zucchini Pasta Sauce For Kids	2.9 %
Coles	Tuna Pasta Bake	3.0 %
Global Organics	Tomato Passata Rustica	3.0 %
Leggo's	Creamy Mushroom Pasta Sauce	3.0 %
TRADITIONAL		
Chicken Tonight	Creamy Mushroom Simmer Sauce	0.9 %
Simmer Sensations	Classic Stroganoff Simmer Sauce	1.1 %
Stroganoff Tonight	Creamy Hungarian Stroganoff Simmer Sauce	1.1 %
Chicken Tonight	Country French White Wine Simmer Sauce	1.4 %
Chicken Tonight	Cheese & Bacon Simmer Sauce	1.6 %
Chicken Tonight	Creamy Chicken & Leek Cooking Sauce	1.8 %
Celebrate Health	Honey Mustard Chicken	2.0 %
Chicken Tonight	Traditional Farmhouse Chicken Cooking Sauce	2.1 %
Chicken Tonight	Vegetable Curry Simmer Sauce	2.8 %
OTHER		
Ozganics	Moroccan Spicy Lamb Tagine Simmer Sauce	2.7 %

Breakfast Cereals

I've presented this list in two formats so you can browse by sugar content or brand.

Breakfast Cereals - by sugar content

Brand	Label	% Sugar
Coles	Organic Instant Rolled Oats	0.0 %
Coles	Organic Traditional Rolled Oats	0.0 %
Coles	Wholegrain Rolled Oats	0.0 %
Nature First Organic	Instant Oats	0.0 %
Nature First Organic	Traditional Rolled Oats	0.0 %
Pureharvest	Organic Rolled Oats	0.0 %
Red Tractor	Instant Oats Omega 3	0.1 %
Golden Vale	Quick Oats	0.2 %
Good Morning Cereals	Buckwheat Puffs	0.2 %
Good Morning Cereals	Multi Puffs	0.2 %
Good Morning Cereals	Millet Puffs	0.4 %
Uncle Tobys	VitaBrits	0.4 %
Uncle Tobys	VitaBrits Weeties	0.4 %
Bob's Red Mill	Mighty Tasty Multi Grain Porridge	0.5 %
Bob's Red Mill	Organic Creamy Buckwheat Whole Grain Hot Cereal	0.5 %
Bob's Red Mill	Organic Creamy Rice Brown Rice Farina Hot Cereal	0.5 %
Bob's Red Mill	Organic Oat Bran High Fibre Cereal	0.5 %
Bob's Red Mill	Organic Scottish Oatmeal	0.5 %
Bob's Red Mill	Organic Whole Grain 6 Grain with Flaxseed Hot Cereal	0.5 %

Brand	Label	% Sugar
Freedom Foods	Porridge	0.5 %
Golden Vale	Rolled Oats	0.5 %
Good Morning Cereals	Brown Rice Puffs	0.5 %
Red Tractor	Instant Oats 100 % Australian	0.5 %
Woolworths Macro Organic	Australian Whole Grain Steel Cut Oats	0.5 %
Goodness Superfoods	Traditional Barley + Oats	0.6 %
Real Good Food	Organic Premium Aussie Oats	0.6 %
Carman's	Traditional Australian Super Porridge Oats	0.7 %
Lowan Whole Foods	Wholegrain Rolled Oats	0.7 %
Pureharvest	Organic Quick Cooking Oats	0.7 %
Heartland Harvest	Porridge Blend	0.8 %
Monster Health Food Co	Multigrain Porridge	0.8 %
Red Tractor	Steel-Cut Oats	0.8 %
Sanitarium	Puffed Wheat	0.8 %
Uncle Tobys	OatBrits	0.8 %
Lowan Whole Foods	Rice Flakes	0.9 %
Lowan Whole Foods	Wholegrain Quick Oats	0.9 %
Nature First Organic	Puffed Millet	0.9 %
Abundant Earth	Organic Puffed Corn	1.0 %
Abundant Earth	Organic Puffed Millet	1.0 %
Abundant Earth	Puffed Corn	1.0 %
Abundant Earth	Puffed Millet	1.0 %
Bob's Red Mill	10 Grain Pride of the Mill Hot Cereal	1.0 %
Bob's Red Mill	Whole Grain Steel Cut Oats	1.0 %

Brand	Label	% Sugar
Nature First Breakfast	Rice Crisps	1.0 %
Quaker Oats	Traditional Oats	1.0 %
Red Tractor	Instant Oats Natural Protein	1.0 %
Uncle Tobys	Quick Oats	1.0 %
Uncle Tobys	Quick Sachet Oats Original	1.0 %
Uncle Tobys	Steel Cut Oats	1.0 %
Uncle Tobys	Traditional Oats	1.0 %
Abundant Earth	Organic Puffed Rice	1.1 %
Abundant Earth	Puffed Rice	1.1 %
Coles	Smart Buy Quick Oats	1.1 %
Coles	Smart Buy Rolled Oats	1.1 %
Woolworths Macro Organic	Australian Whole Grain Quick Oats	1.1 %
Woolworths Select	Original Wholesome Speedy Oats	1.1 %
Food for Health	Liver Cleansing Muesli	1.2 %
Celebrate Health	Rice & Quinoa Breakfast Cereal	1.3 %
Woolworths Macro Organic	Five Grain Porridge	1.3 %
Woolworths Select	Australian Quick Oats	1.3 %
Woolworths Select	Australian Traditional Oats	1.3 %
Good Morning Cereals	Spelt Puffs	1.4 %
Lowan Whole Foods	Natural Oat Bran	1.4 %
Woolworths Homebrand	Rolled Oats	1.4 %
Woolworths Macro Organic	Australian Traditional Rolled Oats	1.4 %
Coles	Wheat Biscuits	1.5 %

Brand	Label	% Sugar
Good Morning Cereals	Amaranth Puffs	1.5 %
Flax Farms	Gluten Free Porridge	1.6 %
The Muesli	Classic Muesli	1.6 %
Coles	Bran Oats	1.7 %
Coles	Smart Buy Oat Bran	1.7 %
Hubbards	Thank Goodness Gluten Free Cornflakes	1.7 %
Sanitarium	Gluten Free Weet-Bix with Sunflower Seeds & Puffed Rice	1.8 %
Goodness Superfoods	Quick Barley + Oats	1.9 %
Heartland Harvest	Dry Roasted Muesli	1.9 %
Sunsol	Nut Lover's Blend Natural Muesli	1.9 %
The Muesli	Gluten Free Muesli	1.9 %
Woolworths Homebrand	Wheat Biscuits	1.9 %
Bob's Red Mill	Old Fashioned Rolled Oats	2.0 %
Uncle Tobys	Shredded Wheat	2.0 %
Woolworths Homebrand	Natural Bran	2.0 %
Woolworths Macro Organic	Muesli with Mixed Seeds & Nuts	2.1 %
Sanitarium	Gluten Free Weet-Bix	2.2 %
Brookfarm	Gluten Free Porrij	2.3 %
Food for Health	Fibre Cleanse Muesli	2.4 %
Red Tractor	Premium Berry Muesli	2.4 %
Brookfarm	Power Porrij	2.7 %
Golden Vale	Wheat Biscuits	2.8 %
Planet Organic	Gluten Free Porridge	2.9 %

Brand	Label	% Sugar
Sanitarium	Weet-Bix for Kids	2.9 %
Sanitarium	Weet-Bix Organic	2.9 %
Red Tractor	Kids Instant Oats 4 Brains Apple Berry	3.0 %

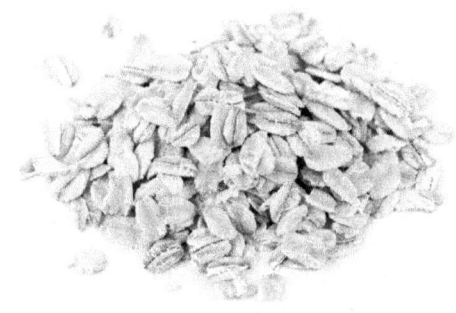

Brand	Label	% Sugar
Abundant Earth	Organic Puffed Corn	1.0 %
	Organic Puffed Millet	1.0 %
	Puffed Corn	1.0 %
	Puffed Millet	1.0 %
	Organic Puffed Rice	1.1 %
	Puffed Rice	1.1 %
Bob's Red Mill	Mighty Tasty Multi Grain Porridge	0.5 %
	Organic Creamy Buckwheat Whole Grain Hot Cereal	0.5 %
	Organic Creamy Rice Brown Rice Farina Hot Cereal	0.5 %
	Organic Oat Bran High Fibre Cereal	0.5 %
	Organic Scottish Oatmeal	0.5 %
	Organic Whole Grain 6 Grain with Flaxseed Hot Cereal	0.5 %
	10 Grain Pride of the Mill Hot Cereal	1.0 %
	Whole Grain Steel Cut Oats	1.0 %
	Old Fashioned Rolled Oats	2.0 %
Brookfarm	Gluten Free Porrij	2.3 %
	Power Porrij	2.7 %
Carman's	Traditional Australian Super Porridge Oats	0.7 %
Celebrate Health	Rice & Quinoa Breakfast Cereal	1.3 %
Coles	Organic Instant Rolled Oats	0.0 %
	Organic Traditional Rolled Oats	0.0 %
	Wholegrain Rolled Oats	0.0 %

Brand	Label	% Sugar
Coles	Smart Buy Quick Oats	1.1 %
	Smart Buy Rolled Oats	1.1 %
	Wheat Biscuits	1.5 %
	Bran Oats	1.7 %
	Smart Buy Oat Bran	1.7 %
Flax Farms	Gluten Free Porridge	1.6 %
Food for Health	Liver Cleansing Muesli	1.2 %
	Fibre Cleanse Muesli	2.4 %
Freedom Foods	Porridge	0.5 %
Golden Vale	Quick Oats	0.2 %
	Rolled Oats	0.5 %
	Wheat Biscuits	2.8 %
Good Morning Cereals	Buckwheat Puffs	0.2 %
	Multi Puffs	0.2 %
	Millet Puffs	0.4 %
	Brown Rice Puffs	0.5 %
	Spelt Puffs	1.4 %
	Amaranth Puffs	1.5 %
Goodness Superfoods	Traditional Barley + Oats	0.6 %
	Quick Barley + Oats	1.9 %
Heartland Harvest	Porridge Blend	0.8 %
	Dry Roasted Muesli	1.9 %
Hubbards	Thank Goodness Gluten Free Cornflakes	1.7 %

Brand	Label	% Sugar
Lowan Whole Foods	Wholegrain Rolled Oats	0.7 %
	Rice Flakes	0.9 %
	Wholegrain Quick Oats	0.9 %
	Natural Oat Bran	1.4 %
Monster Health Food Co	Multigrain Porridge	0.8 %
Nature First Breakfast	Rice Crisps	1.0 %
Nature First Organic	Instant Oats	0.0 %
	Traditional Rolled Oats	0.0 %
	Puffed Millet	0.9 %
Planet Organic	Gluten Free Porridge	2.9 %
Pureharvest	Organic Rolled Oats	0.0 %
	Organic Quick Cooking Oats	0.7 %
Quaker Oats	Traditional Oats	1.0 %
Real Good Food	Organic Premium Aussie Oats	0.6 %
Red Tractor	Instant Oats Omega 3	0.1 %
	Instant Oats 100 % Australian	0.5 %
	Steel-Cut Oats	0.8 %
	Instant Oats Natural Protein	1.0 %
	Premium Berry Muesli	2.4 %
	Kids Instant Oats 4 Brains Apple Berry	3.0 %
Sanitarium	Puffed Wheat	0.8 %
	Gluten Free Weet-Bix with Sunflower Seeds & Puffed Rice	1.8 %

Brand	Label	% Sugar
Sanitarium	Gluten Free Weet-Bix	2.2 %
	Weet-Bix for Kids	2.9 %
	Weet-Bix Organic	2.9 %
Sunsol	Nut Lover's Blend Natural Muesli	1.9 %
The Muesli	Classic Muesli	1.6 %
	Gluten Free Muesli	1.9 %
Uncle Tobys	VitaBrits	0.4 %
	VitaBrits Weeties	0.4 %
	OatBrits	0.8 %
	Quick Oats	1.0 %
	Quick Sachet Oats Original	1.0 %
	Steel Cut Oats	1.0 %
	Traditional Oats	1.0 %
	Shredded Wheat	2.0 %
Woolworths Homebrand	Rolled Oats	1.4 %
	Wheat Biscuits	1.9 %
	Natural Bran	2.0 %
Woolworths Macro Organic	Australian Whole Grain Steel Cut Oats	0.5 %
	Australian Whole Grain Quick Oats	1.1 %
	Five Grain Porridge	1.3 %
	Australian Traditional Rolled Oats	1.4 %
	Muesli with Mixed Seeds & Nuts	2.1 %
Woolworths Select	Original Wholesome Speedy Oats	1.1 %
	Australian Quick Oats	1.3 %
	Australian Traditional Oats	1.3 %

Muesli

Muesli eaters like to think they're a bit better than cereal eaters (go on admit it), so for ease of reference, I've created a separate Muesli list.

Brand	% Sugar
Food for Health Life Food The Liver Cleansing Muesli	1.2 %
The Muesli	1.6 %
Real good food Organic fruit free muesli	1.7 %
Heartland Harvest Dry roasted	1.9 %
The Muesli Gluten Free	1.9 %
Sunsol Nut Lover's Blend Natural Muesli	1.9 %
Flip Shelton's Natural Muesli	1.9 %
the one with just nuts and seeds	2.0 %
Woolworths Macro Organic Muesli with Mixed Seeds and Nuts	2.1 %
Food for Health Life Food The Fibre Cleanse Muesli	2.4 %
Red Tractor Premium Berry Muesli	2.4 %

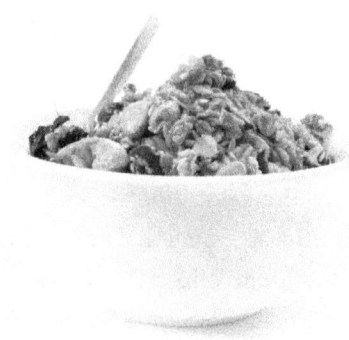

Ice-Cream

You won't be surprised to find that there no store bought ice-creams which satisfy the rule. Even a small bowl (200 g) of the lowest-sugar ice-cream delivers two teaspoons of sugar as well as several artificial sweeteners. And that's not even taking account of the fact that one of the sweeteners (sorbitol) is essentially metabolised as fructose anyway. You'll be pleased to discover that I do provide a great recipe for sugar-free ice-cream in the recipe sections of howmuchsugar.com, in the *Quit Plan Cookbook* and in the *Sweet Poison Quit Plan*. Unfortunately, however, you have to make it yourself; no manufacturer yet makes ice-cream this way.)

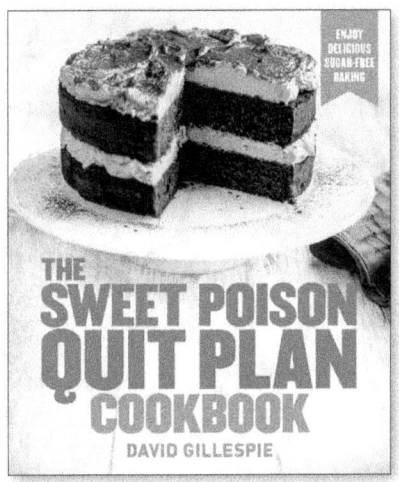
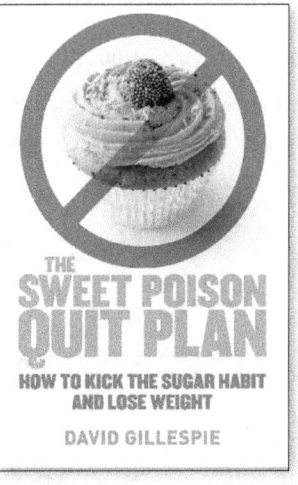

Yoghurts

I've presented this list in two formats so you can browse by sugar content or brand. You'll see that I've also added a column called 'Adjusted Sugar'. This is a calculated amount based on removing the 4.7 grams of lactose that the typical yoghurt contains. Lactose is a galactose molecule joined to a glucose molecule. The galactose molecule is metabolised to glucose by your liver and lactose is therefore essentially pure glucose and fructose free. Lactose does not count towards your 3g per 100g limit.

Yoghurts - by sugar content

Brand	Label	% Sugar	Adjusted % Sugar
Westhaven	Natural Coconut Milk Yoghurt	0.0 %	0.0 %
Woolworths Gold	Natural Greek Yoghurt	2.3 %	0.0 %
Alpine	Natural Coconut Milk Yoghurt	2.9 %	0.0 %
Woolworths Select	Natural Pot Set Greek Style Yoghurt	3.0 %	0.0 %
Alpine	Passionfruit Coconut Milk Yoghurt	3.2 %	0.0 %
Meredith Dairy	Mediterranean Natural Sheep Milk Yoghurt	3.2 %	0.0 %
B-d Farm Paris Creek	Natural Swiss Style Yogurt	3.3 %	0.0 %
Shaw River	Natural Buffalo Milk Yoghurt	3.4 %	0.0 %
Meredith Dairy	Probiotic Natural Sheep Milk Yoghurt	3.5 %	0.0 %
Caprilac	Natural Goat Yoghurt	3.7 %	0.0 %
B-d Farm Paris Creek	Low Fat Yogurt	3.8 %	0.0 %
Chobani	0 % Plain Greek Yogurt	3.8 %	0.0 %

Brand	Label	% Sugar	Adjusted % Sugar
Chobani	2 % Plain Greek Yogurt	3.8 %	0.0 %
Nestle	Soleil No Fat Vanilla Yoghurt	3.8 %	0.0 %
Caprilac	Berry Delight Goat Yoghurt	3.9 %	0.0 %
Nestle	Greek Style Blueberry Yoghurt	3.9 %	0.0 %
Meredith Dairy	Natural Goat Milk Yoghurt	4.0 %	0.0 %
Nestle	Soleil No Fat Strawberry Yoghurt	4.0 %	0.0 %
Jalna	BioDynamic Organic Whole Milk Yoghourt	4.1 %	0.0 %
Nestle	Soleil No Fat Mixed Berry Yoghurt	4.2 %	0.0 %
Lyttos	Greek Style Pot Set Natural Yogurt 2kg	4.3 %	0.0 %
Nestle	Soleil No Fat Passionfruit Yoghurt	4.3 %	0.0 %
Nestle	Soleil No Fat Tropical Yoghurt	4.4 %	0.0 %
Nestle	Soleil No Fat Black Cherry Yoghurt	4.5 %	0.0 %
Nestle	Soleil No Fat Peach & Mango Yoghurt	4.5 %	0.0 %
Nestle	Greek Style Mango Yoghurt	4.7 %	0.0 %
Schulz Organic Dairy	Organic Natural Yogurt	4.7 %	0.0 %
Westhaven	Goats Milk Natural Yoghurt	4.7 %	0.0 %
Jalna	Greek Natural Yoghourt	4.8 %	0.1 %
Lyttos	Greek Style Pot Set Natural Yogurt 1kg	4.8 %	0.1 %
Black Swan	Detox Greek Style Breakfast Yoghurt	5.0 %	0.3 %
Black Swan	Naturally Sweet Greek Style Breakfast Yoghurt	5.0 %	0.3 %
Yoplait	Formé French Vanilla Yoghurt	5.0 %	0.3 %

Brand	Label	% Sugar	Adjusted % Sugar
B-d Farm Paris Creek	Indulgence Greek Style Yogurt	5.1 %	0.4 %
Tamar Valley	Greek Style Yoghurt	5.2 %	0.5 %
Yoplait	Formé Strawberry Yoghurt	5.2 %	0.5 %
The Margaret River Dairy Company	Creamy Pot Set Greek Style Yoghurt	5.3 %	0.6 %
Yoplait	Formé Raspberry Yoghurt	5.3 %	0.6 %
Black Swan	Naturally Sweet Greek Style No Fat Breakfast Yoghurt	5.4 %	0.7 %
Yoplait	Formé Field Berries Yoghurt	5.4 %	0.7 %
Yoplait	Formé Passionfruit Yoghurt	5.4 %	0.7 %
Jalna	Fat Free Natural Yoghourt	5.5 %	0.8 %
Yoplait	Formé Peach Mango Yoghurt	5.5 %	0.8 %
Yoplait	Formé Tropical Yoghurt	5.5 %	0.8 %
Five:am	Natural No Added Sugar Yoghurt	5.6 %	0.9 %
Jalna	a2 Low Fat Natural Yoghourt	5.6 %	0.9 %
Woolworths Select	Natural Greek Style Yoghurt	5.7 %	1.0 %
Black Swan	No Fat Greek Style Natural Yoghurt	5.9 %	1.2 %
Just Organic	Natural Yogurt	6.0 %	1.3 %
The Margaret River Dairy Company	Creamy Pot Set Natural Yoghurt	6.0 %	1.3 %
Westhaven	Goats Milk Berry Harvest Yoghurt	6.0 %	1.3 %
Gippsland Dairy	Organic Natural Yogurt	6.1 %	1.4 %
Tamar Valley	Light Greek Style Yoghurt	6.1 %	1.4 %

Brand	Label	% Sugar	Adjusted % Sugar
Five:am	Greek Style Yoghurt	6.2 %	1.5 %
Tamar Valley	Natural Yoghurt	6.2 %	1.5 %
Westhaven	Natural Creamy Yoghurt	6.2 %	1.5 %
Woolworths Macro Organic	Greek Style Yoghurt	6.2 %	1.5 %
Kahvecioglu	Natural Yoghurt	6.3 %	1.6 %
Activia	Pure Natural Greek Style Yoghurt	6.5 %	1.8 %
Black Swan	Vanilla Bean Greek Style Natural Yoghurt	6.5 %	1.8 %
Farmers Union	Natural Pot Set Yogurt	6.5 %	1.8 %
Westhaven	Goats Milk Mango Yoghurt	6.5 %	1.8 %
Coles	Natural Pot Set Yoghurt	6.6 %	1.9 %
Jalna	Greek Low Fat Yoghourt	6.7 %	2.0 %
Jalna	Premium Natural Creamy Yoghourt	6.7 %	2.0 %
Pauls	All Natural Original Yoghurt	6.7 %	2.0 %
Tamar Valley	No Added Sugar Greek Style Strawberry Yoghurt	6.7 %	2.0 %
Tamar Valley	No Fat Natural Yoghurt	6.7 %	2.0 %
Pasha	Natural Yoghurt	6.8 %	2.1 %
Tamar Valley	No Added Sugar Greek Style Mixed Berry Yoghurt	6.8 %	2.1 %
Tamar Valley	No Added Sugar Greek Style Raspberry Yoghurt	6.8 %	2.1 %
Farmers Union	Greek Style Natural Yogurt	6.9 %	2.2 %
Pauls	All Natural 99.8 % Fat Free Yoghurt	6.9 %	2.2 %
Lyttos	Greek Style Lite Natural Yogurt	7.0 %	2.3 %

Brand	Label	% Sugar	Adjusted % Sugar
Tamar Valley	No Added Sugar Greek Style Citrus Cheesecake Yoghurt	7.0 %	2.3 %
Eat.	Natural (Unsweetened) Organic Yoghurt	7.1 %	2.4 %
Moo	Dahi Indian-Style Yoghurt	7.1 %	2.4 %
Tamar Valley	No Added Sugar Greek Style Passionfruit Yoghurt	7.1 %	2.4 %
Westhaven	Berry Temptation Creamy Yoghurt	7.2 %	2.5 %
Westhaven	Boysenberry Creamy Yoghurt	7.2 %	2.5 %
Westhaven	Mango Creamy Yoghurt	7.2 %	2.5 %
Westhaven	Strawberry Creamy Yoghurt	7.2 %	2.5 %
Black Swan	Traditional Greek Style Natural Yoghurt	7.3 %	2.6 %
Tamar Valley	No Added Sugar Greek Style Mango Yoghurt	7.4 %	2.7 %
Tamar Valley	No Added Sugar Greek Style Plain Yoghurt	7.4 %	2.7 %
Vaalia	Low Fat Natural Yoghurt	7.4 %	2.7 %

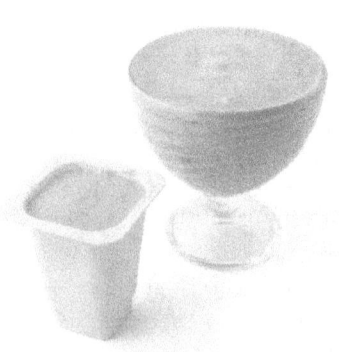

Brand	Label	% Sugar	Adjusted % Sugar
Activia	Pure Natural Greek Style Yoghurt	6.5 %	1.8 %
Alpine	Natural Coconut Milk Yoghurt	2.9 %	0.0 %
	Passionfruit Coconut Milk Yoghurt	3.2 %	0.0 %
B-d Farm Paris Creek	Natural Swiss Style Yogurt	3.3 %	0.0 %
	Low Fat Yogurt	3.8 %	0.0 %
	Indulgence Greek Style Yogurt	5.1 %	0.4 %
Black Swan	Detox Greek Style Breakfast Yoghurt	5.0 %	0.3 %
	Naturally Sweet Greek Style Breakfast Yoghurt	5.0 %	0.3 %
	Naturally Sweet Greek Style No Fat Breakfast Yoghurt	5.4 %	0.7 %
	No Fat Greek Style Natural Yoghurt	5.9 %	1.2 %
	Vanilla Bean Greek Style Natural Yoghurt	6.5 %	1.8 %
	Traditional Greek Style Natural Yoghurt	7.3 %	2.6 %
Caprilac	Natural Goat Yoghurt	3.7 %	0.0 %
	Berry Delight Goat Yoghurt	3.9 %	0.0 %
Chobani	0 % Plain Greek Yogurt	3.8 %	0.0 %
	2 % Plain Greek Yogurt	3.8 %	0.0 %
Coles	Natural Pot Set Yoghurt	6.6 %	1.9 %
Eat.	Natural (Unsweetened) Organic Yoghurt	7.1 %	2.4 %
Farmers Union	Natural Pot Set Yogurt	6.5 %	1.8 %
	Greek Style Natural Yogurt	6.9 %	2.2 %
Five:am	Natural No Added Sugar Yoghurt	5.6 %	0.9 %

Brand	Label	% Sugar	Adjusted % Sugar
Five:am	Greek Style Yoghurt	6.2 %	1.5 %
Gippsland Dairy	Organic Natural Yogurt	6.1 %	1.4 %
Jalna	BioDynamic Organic Whole Milk Yoghourt	4.1 %	0.0 %
	Greek Natural Yoghourt	4.8 %	0.1 %
	Fat Free Natural Yoghourt	5.5 %	0.8 %
	a2 Low Fat Natural Yoghourt	5.6 %	0.9 %
	Greek Low Fat Yoghourt	6.7 %	2.0 %
	Premium Natural Creamy Yoghourt	6.7 %	2.0 %
Just Organic	Natural Yogurt	6.0 %	1.3 %
Kahvecioglu	Natural Yoghurt	6.3 %	1.6 %
Lyttos	Greek Style Pot Set Natural Yogurt 2kg	4.3 %	0.0 %
	Greek Style Pot Set Natural Yogurt 1kg	4.8 %	0.1 %
	Greek Style Lite Natural Yogurt	7.0 %	2.3 %
Meredith Dairy	Mediterranean Natural Sheep Milk Yoghurt	3.2 %	0.0 %
	Probiotic Natural Sheep Milk Yoghurt	3.5 %	0.0 %
	Natural Goat Milk Yoghurt	4.0 %	0.0 %
Moo	Dahi Indian-Style Yoghurt	7.1 %	2.4 %
Nestle	Soleil No Fat Vanilla Yoghurt	3.8 %	0.0 %
	Greek Style Blueberry Yoghurt	3.9 %	0.0 %
	Soleil No Fat Strawberry Yoghurt	4.0 %	0.0 %
	Soleil No Fat Mixed Berry Yoghurt	4.2 %	0.0 %
	Soleil No Fat Passionfruit Yoghurt	4.3 %	0.0 %

Brand	Label	% Sugar	Adjusted % Sugar
Nestle	Soleil No Fat Tropical Yoghurt	4.4 %	0.0 %
	Soleil No Fat Black Cherry Yoghurt	4.5 %	0.0 %
	Soleil No Fat Peach & Mango Yoghurt	4.5 %	0.0 %
	Greek Style Mango Yoghurt	4.7 %	0.0 %
Pasha	Natural Yoghurt	6.8 %	2.1 %
Pauls	All Natural Original Yoghurt	6.7 %	2.0 %
	All Natural 99.8 % Fat Free Yoghurt	6.9 %	2.2 %
Schulz Organic Dairy	Organic Natural Yogurt	4.7 %	0.0 %
Shaw River	Natural Buffalo Milk Yoghurt	3.4 %	0.0 %
Tamar Valley	Greek Style Yoghurt	5.2 %	0.5 %
	Light Greek Style Yoghurt	6.1 %	1.4 %
	Natural Yoghurt	6.2 %	1.5 %
	No Added Sugar Greek Style Strawberry Yoghurt	6.7 %	2.0 %
	No Fat Natural Yoghurt	6.7 %	2.0 %
	No Added Sugar Greek Style Mixed Berry Yoghurt	6.8 %	2.1 %
	No Added Sugar Greek Style Raspberry Yoghurt	6.8 %	2.1 %
	No Added Sugar Greek Style Citrus Cheesecake Yoghurt	7.0 %	2.3 %
	No Added Sugar Greek Style Passionfruit Yoghurt	7.1 %	2.4 %
	No Added Sugar Greek Style Mango Yoghurt	7.4 %	2.7 %
Tamar Valley	No Added Sugar Greek Style Plain Yoghurt	7.4 %	2.7 %

Brand	Label	% Sugar	Adjusted % Sugar
The Margaret River Dairy Company	Creamy Pot Set Greek Style Yoghurt	5.3 %	0.6 %
	Creamy Pot Set Natural Yoghurt	6.0 %	1.3 %
Vaalia	Low Fat Natural Yoghurt	7.4 %	2.7 %
Westhaven	Natural Coconut Milk Yoghurt	0.0 %	0.0 %
	Goats Milk Natural Yoghurt	4.7 %	0.0 %
	Goats Milk Berry Harvest Yoghurt	6.0 %	1.3 %
	Natural Creamy Yoghurt	6.2 %	1.5 %
	Goats Milk Mango Yoghurt	6.5 %	1.8 %
	Berry Temptation Creamy Yoghurt	7.2 %	2.5 %
	Boysenberry Creamy Yoghurt	7.2 %	2.5 %
	Mango Creamy Yoghurt	7.2 %	2.5 %
	Strawberry Creamy Yoghurt	7.2 %	2.5 %
Woolworths Gold	Natural Greek Yoghurt	2.3 %	0.0 %
Woolworths Macro Organic	Greek Style Yoghurt	6.2 %	1.5 %
Woolworths Select	Natural Pot Set Greek Style Yoghurt	3.0 %	0.0 %
	Natural Greek Style Yoghurt	5.7 %	1.0 %
Yoplait	Formé French Vanilla Yoghurt	5.0 %	0.3 %
	Formé Strawberry Yoghurt	5.2 %	0.5 %
	Formé Raspberry Yoghurt	5.3 %	0.6 %
	Formé Field Berries Yoghurt	5.4 %	0.7 %
	Formé Passionfruit Yoghurt	5.4 %	0.7 %
	Formé Peach Mango Yoghurt	5.5 %	0.8 %
	Formé Tropical Yoghurt	5.5 %	0.8 %

Breads

I've presented this list in two formats so you can browse by sugar content or brand. Almost all of the supermarket brands of bread contain canola oil or another seed oil. If you are concerned about seed oil content then you will need to read the labels carefully. *Avoid any that say they contain 'Vegetable Oil'*

Breads - by sugar content

Brand	Type	% Sugar
Baker's Delight	White Spelt Bread	0.1 %
Bakers Life	Artisan Style Pane Di Casa	0.1 %
Bakers Life	English Muffins	0.1 %
Bakers Life	White Wraps	0.1 %
Bakers Life	Wholegrain Wraps	0.1 %
Bill's Organic	100 % Spelt Sourdough	0.1 %
Bill's Organic	Ancient Grains Activated Super Seeds Sourdough	0.1 %
Bakers Life	Bakehouse White Bread	0.2 %
Dovedale	Rice Chia Bread	0.2 %
Healthybake	Classic White Organic Bread	0.2 %
Bill's Organic	100 % Wholemeal Sourdough	0.3 %
Bill's Organic	Activated 7 Seeds Multigrain Sourdough	0.3 %
Bill's Organic	Ancient Grains Power Protein Sourdough	0.3 %
Edward's Sourdough	Organic Khorasan Chia Grain	0.3 %
Goodness Superfoods	Better for U Barley Wraps	0.3 %
Edward's Sourdough	Dark Rye	0.4 %

Brand	Type	% Sugar
Edward's Sourdough	Light Rye	0.4 %
Edward's Sourdough	Organic Purple Spelt	0.4 %
Lichtenstein's Bakehouse	Wholemeal Sourdough Spelt Bread	0.4 %
Vitality Bakehouse	Homestyle Rye Grid Sourdough	0.4 %
Woolworths Select	Wholemeal Sandwich Pockets	0.4 %
Coles Simply	Gluten Free White Wraps	0.5 %
Dovedale	High Fibre Chia Bread	0.5 %
Healthybake	Five Seed Organic Bread	0.5 %
MEB Foods	Wholemeal Ancient Grains & Seeds Pita Bread	0.5 %
Country Life Bakery	Reduced Wheat Country Grain & Organic Rye Bread	0.5 %
Bakers Life	Artisan Style Country Seed Sourdough	0.6 %
Dovedale	Rye Chia Bread	0.6 %
Edward's Sourdough	Soy Linseed	0.6 %
Edward's Sourdough	Spelt Wholemeal	0.6 %
Bakers Life	Lebanese Wholemeal Flat Bread	0.7 %
Bill's Organic	Medium Rye Sourdough	0.7 %
Edward's Sourdough	Organic 7 Grain	0.7 %
Edward's Sourdough	Organic Rye	0.7 %
Edward's Sourdough	Spelt Wholemeal Grain	0.7 %
Schwob's	Bread Plus Kibbled Rye	0.7 %
Bakers Life	Sunny Crumpets	0.8 %
Edward's Sourdough	Organic Barley Oat	0.8 %
Wattle Valley	Lite White Soft Wraps	0.8 %
MEB Foods	Garlic Afghan Bread	0.9 %

Brand	Type	% Sugar
PureBred	Multigrain Farmhouse Loaf	0.9 %
Schar	Meisterbackers Vital Bread	0.9 %
Alpine Breads	Super Natural Protein Rolls	1.0 %
Golden	Crumpets	1.0 %
Golden	Wholemeal Crumpets	1.0 %
Lichtenstein's Bakehouse	Country Loaf	1.0 %
Nature First Organic	Whole Rye Bread with Flax Seeds	1.0 %
PureBred	Seeded Wholegrain Sandwich Rolls	1.0 %
Toscano	Mini Panini	1.0 %
Dovedale	Multiseed Chia Bread	1.1 %
Baker's Delight	Hi-Fibre Low-GI White Loafs	1.2 %
Baker's Delight	High Fibre Tiger Loaf	1.2 %
Country Grainstore	Organic Rye Flour Wraps	1.2 %
Helga's	Traditional White Wraps	1.2 %
MEB Foods	Turkish Pide Bread	1.2 %
MEB Foods	Turkish Rolls	1.2 %
Mountain Bread	Spelt Wraps	1.2 %
Zehnder	White Potato Bread	1.2 %
Baker's Delight	Chia Omega-3 White Bread	1.3 %
Baker's Delight	Fresh Pizza Base	1.3 %
Baker's Delight	Hi-Fibre Low-GI White Roll	1.3 %
Baker's Delight	High Fibre Tiger Small Loaf	1.3 %
Baker's Delight	White Table Roll	1.3 %
Coles	White Soft Wraps	1.3 %
Dovedale	Tiger White Bread	1.3 %

Brand	Type	% Sugar
PureBred	Hamburger Buns	1.3 %
PureBred	White Farmhouse Loaf	1.3 %
Wattle Valley	Sourdough Soft Wraps	1.3 %
Baker's Delight	Hi-Fibre Low-GI White Dinner Rolls	1.4 %
Baker's Delight	White Loafs	1.4 %
Baker's Delight	White Rolls	1.4 %
Bakers Life	Lebanese White Flat Bread	1.4 %
Bakers Life	Multigrain Sandwich Bread	1.4 %
Lawson's	Homestead Seed & Grain Bread	1.4 %
MEB Foods	Khobz White Lite Lebanese Bread	1.4 %
MEB Foods	Souvlaki & Pizza Lite Pittes	1.4 %
PureBred	Supersoft White Sandwich Rolls	1.4 %
Woolworths Select	Crumpets	1.4 %
Zehnder	Soy Linseed Bread	1.4 %
Baker's Delight	Herb and Garlic Sub Roll	1.5 %
Baker's Delight	High Fibre Tiger Roll	1.5 %
Baker's Delight	Parmesan Sub Roll	1.5 %
Baker's Delight	White Bread Stick	1.5 %
Baker's Delight	White Sub Roll	1.5 %
Helga's	Mixed Grain Wraps	1.5 %
MEB Foods	Khobz Rye Lite Lebanese Bread	1.5 %
Mountain Bread	Chia Wraps	1.5 %
Wonder White	Hi Fibre Soft Wraps	1.5 %
Baker's Delight	White Dinner Rolls	1.6 %
Baker's Delight	White Tiger Farmers Loaf	1.6 %

Brand	Type	% Sugar
Coles	Wholemeal & Grain Soft Wraps	1.6 %
Dovedale	Rice Chia Buns	1.6 %
Helga's	Schinkenbrot Bread	1.6 %
Lawson's	Settlers Grain Bread	1.6 %
MEB Foods	Khobz Wholemeal Lebanese Bread	1.6 %
MEB Foods	Wholemeal Lite Family Pita	1.6 %
MEB Foods	Wholemeal Lite Pocket Pita	1.6 %
MEB Foods	Wholemeal Pita Bread	1.6 %
Mestemacher	Organic Flaxseed Bread	1.6 %
PureBred	Chia Seed Loaf	1.6 %
Supreme Quality Foods	Garlic Naan Bread	1.6 %
Tip Top	Multigrain English Muffins	1.6 %
Alpine Breads	Rye Grain Bread	1.7 %
Baker's Delight	White Tiger Roll	1.7 %
Coles Simply	Gluten Free Chia & Seed Bread	1.7 %
Helga's	Black Rye Bread	1.7 %
Mestemacher	Pumpkin Seed Bread	1.7 %
Mighty Soft	Multigrain Sandwich Bread	1.7 %
Burgen	Rye Bread	1.8 %
Coles	Lite White Soft Wraps	1.8 %
Livwell	Crumpets	1.8 %
Mestemacher	Organic Three Grain Bread	1.8 %
Mountain Bread	Oat Wraps	1.8 %
Mountain Bread	White Wraps	1.8 %
Toscano	Bruschettina	1.8 %

Brand	Type	% Sugar
Wattle Valley	Rye Bread Soft Wraps	1.8 %
Wattle Valley	Wheat & Rye Soft Wraps	1.8 %
Wattle Valley	Wholegrain Soft Wraps	1.8 %
Maharajah's Choice	Garlic & Coriander Naan	1.9 %
Mighty Soft	Wholemeal Sandwich Bread	1.9 %
Mountain Bread	Oregano Flavoured Wraps	1.9 %
Schwob's	Dark Rye Cob	1.9 %
Tip Top	9 Grain Wholemeal Bread	1.9 %
Vitastic	Wholemeal Sorj Wraps	1.9 %
Wonder White	Smooth Wholemeal Soft Wraps	1.9 %
Woolworths Homebrand	Multigrain Sandwich Bread	1.9 %
Zehnder	Multiseed Bread Rolls	1.9 %
Zehnder	White Bread Rolls	1.9 %
Coles	Multigrain Round Rolls	2.0 %
Country Grainstore	Organic Spelt Flour Wraps	2.0 %
Country Grainstore	Organic Wheat Flour Wraps	2.0 %
Country Grainstore	Wraps Delight	2.0 %
Grainburg	Rye Bread	2.0 %
Helga's	Sweet & Sour Rye with Caraway Bread	2.0 %
Maharajah's Choice	Plain Naan	2.0 %
Mighty Soft	Wholemeal Muffins	2.0 %
Mission	White Corn Tortillas	2.0 %
Schwob's	Bread Plus Soy & Linseed	2.0 %
Tip Top	Wholemeal English Muffins	2.0 %
Toscano	Pizza Bruschettina	2.0 %

Brand	Type	% Sugar
True Foods	Garlic Naans	2.0 %
Alpine Breads	Spelt & Barley Bread	2.1 %
Alpine Breads	Super Natural Spelt Bread	2.1 %
Bakers Life	Turkish Pide Bread	2.1 %
Bakers Life	Turkish Pide Rolls	2.1 %
Helga's	Soy & Linseed Bread	2.1 %
Lawson's	Original White Bread	2.1 %
Maharajah's Choice	Masala Naan	2.1 %
MEB Foods	White Lite Pocket Pita	2.1 %
MEB Foods	White Pita Bread	2.1 %
Mountain Bread	Rice Wraps	2.1 %
Tip Top	9 Grain Pumpkin Seed Bread	2.1 %
Woolworths	Free From Gluten White Corn Tortillas	2.1 %
Zehnder	Olive Bread	2.1 %
Burgen	Pumpkin Seeds Bread	2.2 %
Buttercup	Country Split Wholemeal Bread	2.2 %
Mestemacher	Organic Rye & Spelt Bread	2.2 %
Old Time Bakery	Certified Organic Gluten Free Wraps	2.2 %
Tip Top	9 Grain Original Bread	2.2 %
Classic Indian	Traditional Roti Bread	2.3 %
Coles	Wholemeal Round Rolls	2.3 %
Helga's	Quinoa & Flaxseed Bread	2.3 %
MEB Foods	White Flat Bread	2.3 %
Mountain Bread	Natural Wraps	2.3 %
Mountain Bread	Rye Wraps	2.3 %

Brand	Type	% Sugar
Mountain Bread	White Wheat Wraps	2.3 %
True Foods	Traditional Roti Wraps	2.3 %
Alpine Breads	Spelt & Sprouted Grains Bread	2.4 %
Atta Foods	Traditional Chapatti	2.4 %
Australia's Own Organic	Multigrain Organic Wraps	2.4 %
Bakers Life	Artisan Style Sourdough	2.4 %
Bakers Life	Grain Wise Original Bread	2.4 %
Burgen	Soy & Linseed Bread	2.4 %
Burgen	Wholegrain & Oats Bread	2.4 %
Burgen	Wholemeal & Seeds Bread	2.4 %
Classic Indian	Garlic Roti Bread	2.4 %
Coles Smart Buy	Wholemeal Sandwich Bread	2.4 %
Country Grainstore	Vienna-Rye Bread	2.4 %
Flinder's Bread	Dark Rye Bread	2.4 %
Helga's	Pumpkin Seed & Grain	2.4 %
Helga's	Traditional Wholemeal Bread	2.4 %
Mission	Chia Wraps	2.4 %
Mountain Bread	Wheat Wraps	2.4 %
Natureen	Rye Bread	2.4 %
Tip Top	Original English Muffins	2.4 %
Tip Top	Sunblest White Sandwich Bread	2.4 %
Tip Top	Sunblest White Thick Bread	2.4 %
Woolworths Select	Mixed Wholegrain Sandwich Bread	2.4 %
Alpine Breads	Tuscany Grain Bread	2.5 %
Atlantic Bakery	Dark Rye Bread	2.5 %

Brand	Type	% Sugar
Coles	Wholemeal Sandwich Bread	2.5 %
Helga's	Light Rye	2.5 %
Helga's	Lower Carb 5 Seeds Bread	2.5 %
MEB Foods	Wholemeal Flat Bread	2.5 %
Mission	Red Quinoa Wraps	2.5 %
Supreme Quality Foods	Fresh Roti Original	2.5 %
Tip Top	Sunblest Multigrain Sandwich Bread	2.5 %
Tip Top	Sunblest Multigrain Thick Bread	2.5 %
Wonder White	Wholemeal + Iron Sandwich Bread	2.5 %
Zehnder	Rice Bread	2.5 %
Australia's Own Organic	Quinoa Organic Wraps	2.6 %
Bakers Life	Bakehouse Mixed Grains Bread	2.6 %
Bakers Life	Wholemeal Sandwich Bread	2.6 %
Buttercup	Country Split White Bread	2.6 %
Coles	White Long Rolls	2.6 %
Coles	White Round Rolls	2.6 %
Globe's	Traditional Chapati Wraps	2.6 %
Helga's	Lower Carb Wholemeal & Seed Bread	2.6 %
Mestemacher	Organic Sunflower Seed Bread	2.6 %
Mountain Bread	Light Spinach Wraps	2.6 %
Mountain Bread	Tomato & Basil Flavoured Wraps	2.6 %
Schwob's	Bread Plus Roasted Seed	2.6 %
Atlantic Bakery	Karl's Light Rye Bread	2.7 %
Bakers Life	Bakehouse Wholemeal Bread	2.7 %

Brand	Type	% Sugar
Flinder's Bread	Sour Dough Rye Bread	2.7 %
Golden	Crumpets with Oats	2.7 %
Supreme Quality Foods	Fresh Roti with Pepper	2.7 %
Tip Top	9 Grain 9 Seeds Bread	2.7 %
Vitastic	Rye Sorj Wraps	2.7 %
Woolworths Select	English Muffins	2.7 %
Woolworths Select	White Sandwich Bread	2.7 %
Coles	English Muffins	2.8 %
Coles	Multigrain Sandwich Bread	2.8 %
Coles	White Sandwich Bread	2.8 %
Coles	White Toast Bread	2.8 %
Country Life Bakery	Reduced Wheat Organic Rye Bread	2.8 %
Has No...	Gluten Free Six Seeds Bread	2.8 %
Molenberg	12 Grains & Seeds Bread	2.8 %
Schwob's	Bread Plus Whole Grain	2.8 %
Taylor's	Wholemeal Bread	2.8 %
Alpine Breads	Sour Rye Bread	2.9 %
Atlantic Bakery	Hausbrot Loaf with Caraway Seeds	2.9 %
Bakers Life	Viva Plus High Fibre White Bread	2.9 %
Bakers Life	Viva Plus Smooth Wholemeal Bread	2.9 %
Coles Smart Buy	Multigrain Sandwich Bread	2.9 %
Coles Smart Buy	White Toast Bread	2.9 %
Grandma Moses	Seed Bread	2.9 %
Has No...	Gluten Free White Bread	2.9 %

Brand	Type	% Sugar
Mountain Bread	Barley Wraps	2.9 %
Mountain Bread	Corn Wraps	2.9 %
Bakers Life	Bakehouse Soy & Linseed Bread	3.0 %
Bakers Life	Bakehouse Traditional Rye Bread	3.0 %
Bakers Life	Super Soft White Bread	3.0 %
Bazaar	Greek Yiros	3.0 %
Bazaar	White Turkish Pide	3.0 %
Bazaar	White Turkish Rolls	3.0 %
Bazaar	Wholemeal Lebanese Breads	3.0 %
Bazaar	Wholemeal Pita Pockets	3.0 %
Coles	Hamburger Rolls	3.0 %
Coles Smart Buy	White Sandwich Bread	3.0 %
Helga's	Lower Carb Sunflower & Golden Linseed Bread	3.0 %
Helga's	Mixed Grain Bread	3.0 %
Helga's	Traditional White Bread	3.0 %
Nature First Organic	Multigrain Bread	3.0 %
Nature First Organic	Pumpernickel Bread	3.0 %
Nature First Organic	Whole Rye Bread	3.0 %
Nature First Organic	Whole Rye Bread with Sunflower Seeds	3.0 %
Supreme Quality Foods	Fresh Paratha Original	3.0 %
Supreme Quality Foods	Fresh Roti with Fenugreek	3.0 %
Tip Top	Sunblest Wholemeal Sandwich Bread	3.0 %
Tip Top	Sunblest Wholemeal Thick Bread	3.0 %

Brand	Type	% Sugar
Tip Top	The One White Sandwich Bread	3.0 %
Tip Top	The One White Toast Bread	3.0 %
Wonder White	Hi Fibre Sandwich Bread	3.0 %
Wonder White	Hi Fibre Toast Bread	3.0 %
Wonder White	Vitamins & Minerals Sandwich Bread	3.0 %
Wonder White	Vitamins & Minerals Toast Bread	3.0 %
Woolworths Select	Smooth Wholemeal Sandwich Bread	3.0 %

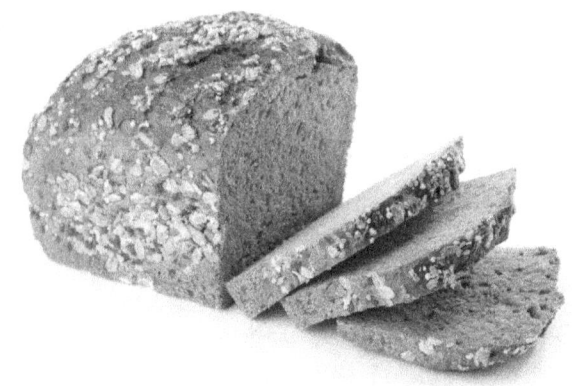

Breads - by brand

Brand	Type	% Sugar
Alpine Breads	Super Natural Protein Rolls	1.0 %
	Rye Grain Bread	1.7 %
	Spelt & Barley Bread	2.1 %
	Super Natural Spelt Bread	2.1 %
	Spelt & Sprouted Grains Bread	2.4 %
	Tuscany Grain Bread	2.5 %
	Sour Rye Bread	2.9 %
Atlantic Bakery	Dark Rye Bread	2.5 %
	Karl's Light Rye Bread	2.7 %
	Hausbrot Loaf with Caraway Seeds	2.9 %
Atta Foods	Traditional Chapatti	2.4 %
Australia's Own Organic	Multigrain Organic Wraps	2.4 %
	Quinoa Organic Wraps	2.6 %
Baker's Delight	White Spelt Bread	0.1 %
	Hi-Fibre Low-GI White Loafs	1.2 %
	High Fibre Tiger Loaf	1.2 %
	Chia Omega-3 White Bread	1.3 %
	Fresh Pizza Base	1.3 %
	Hi-Fibre Low-GI White Roll	1.3 %
	High Fibre Tiger Small Loaf	1.3 %
	White Table Roll	1.3 %
	Hi-Fibre Low-GI White Dinner Rolls	1.4 %
	White Loafs	1.4 %
	White Rolls	1.4 %
	Herb and Garlic Sub Roll	1.5 %

Brand	Type	% Sugar
Baker's Delight	High Fibre Tiger Roll	1.5 %
	Parmesan Sub Roll	1.5 %
	White Bread Stick	1.5 %
	White Sub Roll	1.5 %
	White Dinner Rolls	1.6 %
	White Tiger Farmers Loaf	1.6 %
	White Tiger Roll	1.7 %
Bakers Life	Artisan Style Pane Di Casa	0.1 %
	English Muffins	0.1 %
	White Wraps	0.1 %
	Wholegrain Wraps	0.1 %
	Bakehouse White Bread	0.2 %
	Artisan Style Country Seed Sourdough	0.6 %
	Lebanese Wholemeal Flat Bread	0.7 %
	Sunny Crumpets	0.8 %
	Lebanese White Flat Bread	1.4 %
	Multigrain Sandwich Bread	1.4 %
	Turkish Pide Bread	2.1 %
	Turkish Pide Rolls	2.1 %
	Artisan Style Sourdough	2.4 %
	Grain Wise Original Bread	2.4 %
	Bakehouse Mixed Grains Bread	2.6 %
	Wholemeal Sandwich Bread	2.6 %
	Bakehouse Wholemeal Bread	2.7 %
	Viva Plus High Fibre White Bread	2.9 %

Brand	Type	% Sugar
Bakers Life	Viva Plus Smooth Wholemeal Bread	2.9 %
	Bakehouse Soy & Linseed Bread	3.0 %
	Bakehouse Traditional Rye Bread	3.0 %
	Super Soft White Bread	3.0 %
Bazaar	Greek Yiros	3.0 %
	White Turkish Pide	3.0 %
	White Turkish Rolls	3.0 %
	Wholemeal Lebanese Breads	3.0 %
	Wholemeal Pita Pockets	3.0 %
Bill's Organic	100 % Spelt Sourdough	0.1 %
	Ancient Grains Activated Super Seeds Sourdough	0.1 %
	100 % Wholemeal Sourdough	0.3 %
	Activated 7 Seeds Multigrain Sourdough	0.3 %
	Ancient Grains Power Protein Sourdough	0.3 %
	Medium Rye Sourdough	0.7 %
Burgen	Rye Bread	1.8 %
	Pumpkin Seeds Bread	2.2 %
	Soy & Linseed Bread	2.4 %
	Wholegrain & Oats Bread	2.4 %
	Wholemeal & Seeds Bread	2.4 %
Buttercup	Country Split Wholemeal Bread	2.2 %
	Country Split White Bread	2.6 %
Classic Indian	Traditional Roti Bread	2.3 %
	Garlic Roti Bread	2.4 %

Brand	Type	% Sugar
Coles	White Soft Wraps	1.3 %
	Wholemeal & Grain Soft Wraps	1.6 %
	Lite White Soft Wraps	1.8 %
	Multigrain Round Rolls	2.0 %
	Wholemeal Round Rolls	2.3 %
	Wholemeal Sandwich Bread	2.5 %
	White Long Rolls	2.6 %
	White Round Rolls	2.6 %
	English Muffins	2.8 %
	Multigrain Sandwich Bread	2.8 %
	White Sandwich Bread	2.8 %
	White Toast Bread	2.8 %
	Hamburger Rolls	3.0 %
Coles Simply	Gluten Free White Wraps	0.5 %
	Gluten Free Chia & Seed Bread	1.7 %
Coles Smart Buy	Wholemeal Sandwich Bread	2.4 %
	Multigrain Sandwich Bread	2.9 %
	White Toast Bread	2.9 %
	White Sandwich Bread	3.0 %
Country Grainstore	Organic Rye Flour Wraps	1.2 %
	Organic Spelt Flour Wraps	2.0 %
	Organic Wheat Flour Wraps	2.0 %
	Wraps Delight	2.0 %
	Vienna-Rye Bread	2.4 %
Country Life Bakery	Reduced Wheat Country Grain & Organic Rye Bread	0.5 %

Breads - by brand (continued)

Brand	Type	% Sugar
Country Life Bakery	Reduced Wheat Organic Rye Bread	2.8 %
Dovedale	Rice Chia Bread	0.2 %
	High Fibre Chia Bread	0.5 %
	Rye Chia Bread	0.6 %
	Multiseed Chia Bread	1.1 %
	Tiger White Bread	1.3 %
	Rice Chia Buns	1.6 %
Edward's Sourdough	Organic Khorasan Chia Grain	0.3 %
	Dark Rye	0.4 %
	Light Rye	0.4 %
	Organic Purple Spelt	0.4 %
	Soy Linseed	0.6 %
	Spelt Wholemeal	0.6 %
	Organic 7 Grain	0.7 %
	Organic Rye	0.7 %
	Spelt Wholemeal Grain	0.7 %
	Organic Barley Oat	0.8 %
Flinder's Bread	Dark Rye Bread	2.4 %
	Sour Dough Rye Bread	2.7 %
Globe's	Traditional Chapati Wraps	2.6 %
Golden	Crumpets	1.0 %
	Wholemeal Crumpets	1.0 %
	Crumpets with Oats	2.7 %
Goodness Superfoods	Better for U Barley Wraps	0.3 %
Grainburg	Rye Bread	2.0 %
Grandma Moses	Seed Bread	2.9 %

Brand	Type	% Sugar
Has No...	Gluten Free Six Seeds Bread	2.8 %
	Gluten Free White Bread	2.9 %
Healthybake	Classic White Organic Bread	0.2 %
	Five Seed Organic Bread	0.5 %
Helga's	Traditional White Wraps	1.2 %
	Mixed Grain Wraps	1.5 %
	Schinkenbrot Bread	1.6 %
	Black Rye Bread	1.7 %
	Sweet & Sour Rye with Caraway Bread	2.0 %
	Soy & Linseed Bread	2.1 %
	Quinoa & Flaxseed Bread	2.3 %
	Pumpkin Seed & Grain	2.4 %
	Traditional Wholemeal Bread	2.4 %
	Light Rye	2.5 %
	Lower Carb 5 Seeds Bread	2.5 %
	Lower Carb Wholemeal & Seed Bread	2.6 %
	Lower Carb Sunflower & Golden Linseed Bread	3.0 %
	Mixed Grain Bread	3.0 %
	Traditional White Bread	3.0 %
Lawson's	Homestead Seed & Grain Bread	1.4 %
	Settlers Grain Bread	1.6 %
	Original White Bread	2.1 %
Lichtenstein's Bakehouse	Wholemeal Sourdough Spelt Bread	0.4 %
	Country Loaf	1.0 %

Brand	Type	% Sugar
Livwell	Crumpets	1.8 %
Maharajah's Choice	Garlic & Coriander Naan	1.9 %
	Plain Naan	2.0 %
	Masala Naan	2.1 %
MEB Foods	Wholemeal Ancient Grains & Seeds Pita Bread	0.5 %
	Garlic Afghan Bread	0.9 %
	Turkish Pide Bread	1.2 %
	Turkish Rolls	1.2 %
	Khobz White Lite Lebanese Bread	1.4 %
	Souvlaki & Pizza Lite Pittes	1.4 %
	Khobz Rye Lite Lebanese Bread	1.5 %
	Khobz Wholemeal Lebanese Bread	1.6 %
	Wholemeal Lite Family Pita	1.6 %
	Wholemeal Lite Pocket Pita	1.6 %
	Wholemeal Pita Bread	1.6 %
	White Lite Pocket Pita	2.1 %
	White Pita Bread	2.1 %
	White Flat Bread	2.3 %
	Wholemeal Flat Bread	2.5 %
Mestemacher	Organic Flaxseed Bread	1.6 %
	Pumpkin Seed Bread	1.7 %
	Organic Three Grain Bread	1.8 %
	Organic Rye & Spelt Bread	2.2 %
	Organic Sunflower Seed Bread	2.6 %
Mighty Soft	Multigrain Sandwich Bread	1.7 %

Brand	Type	% Sugar
Mighty Soft	Wholemeal Sandwich Bread	1.9 %
	Wholemeal Muffins	2.0 %
Mission	White Corn Tortillas	2.0 %
	Chia Wraps	2.4 %
	Red Quinoa Wraps	2.5 %
Molenberg	12 Grains & Seeds Bread	2.8 %
Mountain Bread	Spelt Wraps	1.2 %
	Chia Wraps	1.5 %
	Oat Wraps	1.8 %
	White Wraps	1.8 %
	Oregano Flavoured Wraps	1.9 %
	Rice Wraps	2.1 %
	Natural Wraps	2.3 %
	Rye Wraps	2.3 %
	White Wheat Wraps	2.3 %
	Wheat Wraps	2.4 %
	Light Spinach Wraps	2.6 %
	Tomato & Basil Flavoured Wraps	2.6 %
	Barley Wraps	2.9 %
	Corn Wraps	2.9 %
Nature First Organic	Whole Rye Bread with Flax Seeds	1.0 %
	Multigrain Bread	3.0 %
	Pumpernickel Bread	3.0 %
	Whole Rye Bread	3.0 %
	Whole Rye Bread with Sunflower Seeds	3.0 %

Brand	Type	% Sugar
Natureen	Rye Bread	2.4 %
Old Time Bakery	Certified Organic Gluten Free Wraps	2.2 %
PureBred	Multigrain Farmhouse Loaf	0.9 %
PureBred	Seeded Wholegrain Sandwich Rolls	1.0 %
	Hamburger Buns	1.3 %
	White Farmhouse Loaf	1.3 %
	Supersoft White Sandwich Rolls	1.4 %
	Chia Seed Loaf	1.6 %
Schar	Meisterbackers Vital Bread	0.9 %
Schwob's	Bread Plus Kibbled Rye	0.7 %
	Dark Rye Cob	1.9 %
	Bread Plus Soy & Linseed	2.0 %
	Bread Plus Roasted Seed	2.6 %
	Bread Plus Whole Grain	2.8 %
Supreme Quality Foods	Garlic Naan Bread	1.6 %
	Fresh Roti Original	2.5 %
	Fresh Roti with Pepper	2.7 %
	Fresh Paratha Original	3.0 %
	Fresh Roti with Fenugreek	3.0 %
Taylor's	Wholemeal Bread	2.8 %
Tip Top	Multigrain English Muffins	1.6 %
	9 Grain Wholemeal Bread	1.9 %
	Wholemeal English Muffins	2.0 %
	9 Grain Pumpkin Seed Bread	2.1 %
	9 Grain Original Bread	2.2 %

Breads - by brand (continued)

Brand	Type	% Sugar
Tip Top	Original English Muffins	2.4 %
	Sunblest White Sandwich Bread	2.4 %
	Sunblest White Thick Bread	2.4 %
	Sunblest Multigrain Sandwich Bread	2.5 %
	Sunblest Multigrain Thick Bread	2.5 %
	9 Grain 9 Seeds Bread	2.7 %
	Sunblest Wholemeal Sandwich Bread	3.0 %
	Sunblest Wholemeal Thick Bread	3.0 %
	The One White Sandwich Bread	3.0 %
	The One White Toast Bread	3.0 %
Toscano	Mini Panini	1.0 %
	Bruschettina	1.8 %
	Pizza Bruschettina	2.0 %
True Foods	Garlic Naans	2.0 %
	Traditional Roti Wraps	2.3 %
Vitality Bakehouse	Homestyle Rye Grid Sourdough	0.4 %
Vitastic	Wholemeal Sorj Wraps	1.9 %
	Rye Sorj Wraps	2.7 %
Wattle Valley	Lite White Soft Wraps	0.8 %
	Sourdough Soft Wraps	1.3 %
	Rye Bread Soft Wraps	1.8 %
	Wheat & Rye Soft Wraps	1.8 %
	Wholegrain Soft Wraps	1.8 %
Wonder White	Hi Fibre Soft Wraps	1.5 %
	Smooth Wholemeal Soft Wraps	1.9 %

Brand	Type	% Sugar
Wonder White	Wholemeal + Iron Sandwich Bread	2.5 %
	Hi Fibre Sandwich Bread	3.0 %
	Hi Fibre Toast Bread	3.0 %
	Vitamins & Minerals Sandwich Bread	3.0 %
	Vitamins & Minerals Toast Bread	3.0 %
Woolworths	Free From Gluten White Corn Tortillas	2.1 %
Woolworths Homebrand	Multigrain Sandwich Bread	1.9 %
Woolworths Select	Wholemeal Sandwich Pockets	0.4 %
	Crumpets	1.4 %
	Mixed Wholegrain Sandwich Bread	2.4 %
	English Muffins	2.7 %
	White Sandwich Bread	2.7 %
	Smooth Wholemeal Sandwich Bread	3.0 %
Zehnder	White Potato Bread	1.2 %
	Soy Linseed Bread	1.4 %
	Multiseed Bread Rolls	1.9 %
	White Bread Rolls	1.9 %
	Olive Bread	2.1 %
	Rice Bread	2.5 %

Gluten Free Bread

Just to make it a bit easier to see, I've broken out the Gluten Free options below.

Brand	Label	% Sugar
Dovedale	Rice Chia Bread	0.2 %
Coles Simply	Gluten Free White Wraps	0.5 %
PureBred	Multigrain Farmhouse Loaf	0.9 %
PureBred	Seeded Wholegrain Sandwich Rolls	1.0 %
PureBred	Hamburger Buns	1.3 %
PureBred	White Farmhouse Loaf	1.3 %
PureBred	Supersoft White Sandwich Rolls	1.4 %
Dovedale	Rice Chia Buns	1.6 %
PureBred	Chia Seed Loaf	1.6 %
Coles Simply	Gluten Free Chia & Seed Bread	1.7 %
Woolworths	Free From Gluten White Corn Tortillas	2.1 %
Old Time Bakery	Certified Organic Gluten Free Wraps	2.2 %
Has No…	Gluten Free Six Seeds Bread	2.8 %
Has No…	Gluten Free White Bread	2.9%

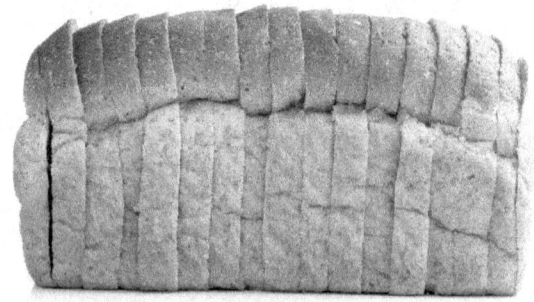

Biscuits

I've presented this list in two formats so you can browse by sugar content or brand. You might notice that all the biscuits in this list are essentially crackers. That's because the lowest sugar sweet biscuit you can get in Australia today is Arnott's Lattice (12 % sugar) and it's a long way outside the 3 percent rule.

Many of these biscuits will contain seed oils. If you are concerned about this, then use the fat reckoner chart available at www.howmuchsugar.com to determine whether your choice is likely to be as low in seed oil as it is in sugar

Biscuits - by sugar content

Brand	Label	% Sugar
Fantastic	Thinner Bite Sesame Black Rice Crackers	0.0 %
Mary's Gone Crackers	Black Pepper Crackers	0.0 %
Mary's Gone Crackers	Caraway Crackers	0.0 %
Mary's Gone Crackers	Herb Crackers	0.0 %
Mary's Gone Crackers	Jalapeno Crackers	0.0 %
Mary's Gone Crackers	Onion Crackers	0.0 %
Mary's Gone Crackers	Original Crackers	0.0 %
Mary's Gone Crackers	Super Seed Crackers	0.0 %
Woolworths Homebrand	Plain Rice Crackers	0.0 %
Arnott's	Original Cracked Pepper	0.1 %
Arnott's	Sesame Water Crackers	0.1 %
Arnott's	Supreme Crackers	0.1 %
Arnott's	Cracked Pepper Water Crackers	0.2 %
Damora	Plain Rice Crackers	0.2 %

Brand	Label	% Sugar
Pureharvest	Organic Thin Corn Cakes	0.2 %
Sakata	Plain Rice Crackers	0.2 %
Always Fresh	Wafer Crackers Roasted Sesame Crisp Bread	0.3 %
Arnott's	Salada Light Original	0.3 %
Arnott's	Shapes Extreme Salt & Vinegar	0.3 %
Melinda's	Natural Crackers	0.3 %
Woolworths Select	Sea Salt Brown Rice Crackers	0.3 %
Arnott's	Salada Original	0.4 %
Arnott's	Shapes Savoury	0.4 %
Pureharvest	Organic Thin Quinoa Rice Cakes	0.4 %
Real Foods	Organic Sesame Corn Thins	0.4 %
Real Foods	Original Corn Thins	0.4 %
Arnott's	Sao Crackers	0.5 %
Arnott's	Vita-Weat Plain Rice Crackers	0.5 %
Belmont Biscuit Co.	Sugar Less Maria Biscuits	0.5 %
Damora	Brown Rice Crackers Original	0.5 %
Gullon	99.5 % Sugar Free Chocolate Chip Cookies	0.5 %
Gullon	99.5 % Sugar Free Digestive Biscuits	0.5 %
Gullon	99.5 % Sugar Free Shortbread Cookies	0.5 %
Orgran	Quinoa Wafer Crackers	0.5 %
Pureharvest	Organic Rice Cakes	0.5 %
Sakata	Sea Salt & Cracked Pepper Rice Crackers	0.5 %
Spiral Foods	Black Sesame Rice Crackers	0.5 %
Spiral Foods	White Sesame Rice Crackers	0.5 %

Brand	Label	% Sugar
Walkers	Fine Oatcakes	0.5 %
Arnott's	Shapes Cheese & Bacon	0.6 %
Arnott's	Vita-Weat Multigrain Rice Crackers	0.6 %
Orgran	Essential Fibre Crispibread	0.6 %
Woolworths Macro Organic	Thick Rice Cakes	0.6 %
Woolworths Select	Original Thin Rice Cakes	0.6 %
Coles	Brown Rice Crackers	0.7 %
Damora	Mini Brown Rice Cakes Original	0.7 %
Orgran	Chia Crispibread	0.7 %
Orgran	Chia Wafer Crackers	0.7 %
Real Foods	Multigrain Corn Thins	0.7 %
Spiral Foods	Tamari Rice Crackers	0.7 %
Always Fresh	Grissini Three Seed & Sea Salt Bread Sticks	0.8 %
Coles	Seeds & Grains Brown Rice Crackers	0.8 %
Real Foods	Soy, Linseed & Chia Corn Thins	0.8 %
Simply Wize	Cheese Deli Wafers	0.8 %
Simply Wize	Poppy Seed & Sea Salt Deli Wafers	0.8 %
Spiral Foods	Vegetable Rice Crackers	0.8 %
SunRice	Original Thin Rice Cakes	0.8 %
SunRice	Wholegrain Brown Rice Original Mini Bites	0.8 %
Arnott's	Cruskits Corn	0.9 %
Arnott's	Cruskits Rice	0.9 %
Arnott's	Salada Multigrain	0.9 %
Arnott's	Shapes BBQ	0.9 %

Brand	Label	% Sugar
Captain's Table	Classic Water Crackers	0.9 %
Captain's Table	Classic Water Crackers	0.9 %
Captain's Table	Cracked Pepper Water Crackers	0.9 %
Captain's Table	Cracked Pepper Water Crackers	0.9 %
Captain's Table	Sesame Seed Water Crackers	0.9 %
Captain's Table	Sesame Seed Water Crackers	0.9 %
Coles	Thin Rice Cakes	0.9 %
Damora	Admiral's Quarters Cracked Pepper Water Crackers	0.9 %
Damora	Admiral's Quarters Original Water Crackers	0.9 %
Damora	Prista Lite Crispbread	0.9 %
Nabisco	Premium 98 % Fat Free Crispbread	0.9 %
Orgran	Corn Crispibread	0.9 %
Orgran	Rice Crispibread	0.9 %
Peckish	BBQ Rice Snackers	0.9 %
Peckish	Brown Rice Crackers	0.9 %
Peckish	Brown Rice Crackers No Salt	0.9 %
Peckish	Cheddar Cheese Rice Crackers	0.9 %
Peckish	Cheese Rice Snackers	0.9 %
Peckish	Herb & Garlic Rice Crackers	0.9 %
Peckish	Original Rice Crackers	0.9 %
Peckish	Pizza Rice Snackers	0.9 %
Peckish	Pizza Supreme Rice Crackers	0.9 %
Peckish	Sea Salt & Vinegar Rice Crackers	0.9 %
Peckish	Sour Cream & Chive Rice Crackers	0.9 %
Peckish	Sour Cream & Chive Rice Snackers	0.9 %

Biscuits - by sugar content (continued)

Brand	Label	% Sugar
Peckish	Sweet Chilli Rice Crackers	0.9 %
Peckish	Tangy BBQ Rice Crackers	0.9 %
Real Foods	Wholegrain Rice Thins	0.9 %
SunRice	Original Thick Rice Cakes	0.9 %
Valley Produce Company	Cracked Black Pepper Crackerthins	0.9 %
Valley Produce Company	Parmesan Cheese Crackerthins	0.9 %
Woolworths Select	Multigrain Brown Rice Crackers	0.9 %
Damora	Brown Rice Crackers Multigrain	1.0 %
Damora	Snackos Barbecue	1.0 %
Roccas Deli	Organic Fine Wafer Crackers	1.0 %
Arnott's	Salada Wholemeal	1.1 %
Fantastic	Goodies Quinoa, Buckwheat, Millet & Amaranth Rice Crackers	1.1 %
Red Tractor	Original Grain Oat Cakes	1.1 %
Damora	Original Thin Rice Cakes	1.1 %
Damora	Snackos Cheese & Bacon	1.1 %
Orgran	Buckwheat Wafer Crackers	1.1 %
Orgran	Quinoa Crispibread	1.1 %
Woolworths Gold	Olive Oil Oatcakes	1.1 %
Arnott's	Cheds Crackers	1.2 %
Simply Fine Food Company	Pepper Lavoche Crispbread	1.2 %
Simply Fine Food Company	Sesame & Poppy Lavoche Crispbread	1.2 %
Walkers	Thick & Crunchy Oatcakes	1.2 %
Arnott's	Savoy Original	1.3 %

Brand	Label	% Sugar
Arnott's	Sesame Wheat Crackers	1.3 %
Fantastic	Salt & Vinegar Rice Crackers	1.3 %
Stonebaker	Garlic, Olive, Rosemary & Parmesan Artisan Baked Pita Bread	1.3 %
Fantastic	Goodies 4 Grains Crackers	1.3 %
Naturally Good	Kasha Toasted Buckwheat Crispbread	1.3 %
Fazer	Crisp Rye	1.4 %
Freelicious	Organic Amaranth & Protein Crispbread	1.4 %
Simply Fine Food Company	Parmesan Lavoche Crispbread	1.4 %
Arnott's	Shapes Extreme Peri Peri Chicken	1.4 %
Arnott's	Shapes Nacho Cheese	1.4 %
Eskal	Original Deli Crackers	1.4 %
Woolworths Gold	Cheese & Seed Straws	1.4 %
Carr's	Garlic & Herbs Table Water Biscuits	1.5 %
Carr's	Sesame Seeds Table Water Biscuits	1.5 %
Damora	Mini Brown Rice Cakes Chicken	1.5 %
Fantastic	Goodies Sesame, Poppy, Sunflower & Mustard Seeds Rice Crackers	1.5 %
Kavli	Crispy Thin Crispbread	1.5 %
Orgran	Premium Multigrain Poppyseed Deli Crackers	1.5 %
Ricci's Bikkies	Garlic, Olive & Parmesan Baked Pita Bread	1.5 %
Ricci's Bikkies	Herbed Baked Pita Bread	1.5 %
Ryvita	Crackerbread	1.5 %
SunRice	Quinoa Rice & Grain Squares	1.5 %

Biscuits - by sugar content (continued)

Brand	Label	% Sugar
SunRice	Wholegrain Brown Rice Chicken Mini Bites	1.5 %
SunRice	Wild Rice Rice & Grain Squares	1.5 %
Woolworths Gold	Cheese Palmiers	1.5 %
Always Fresh	Crustini Olive Oil & Sea Salt Bruschetta Toasts	1.6 %
Arnott's	Shapes Cheddar	1.6 %
Arnott's	Vita-Weat Sesame Crispbread	1.6 %
Carr's	Black Pepper Table Water Biscuits	1.6 %
Carr's	Table Water Biscuits	1.6 %
Damora	Vita Grain Sea Salt & Cracked Pepper Wholegrain Crackers	1.6 %
Finn Crisp	Original Thin Rye Crispbread	1.6 %
SunRice	Buckwheat Rice & Grain Squares	1.6 %
SunRice	Linseed Rice & Grain Squares	1.6 %
Walkers	Highland Oatcakes	1.6 %
Waterthins	Corn Fine Wafer Crackers	1.6 %
Woolworths Gold	Cheese Pretzels	1.6 %
Woolworths Gold	Cheese Twists	1.6 %
Arnott's	Vita-Weat Five Super Seeds Crispbread	1.7 %
Damora	Sanz Family Crackers	1.7 %
Damora	Vita Grain Original Wholegrain Crackers	1.7 %
Fantastic	Crisp'ns Original	1.7 %
Fantastic	Goodies 2 Seeds Crackers	1.7 %
Ricci's Bikkies	Cheese & Chive Baked Pita Bread	1.7 %
Sakata	Wholegrain Original Rice Crackers	1.7 %

Brand	Label	% Sugar
SunRice	Wholegrain Brown Rice Salt & Vinegar Mini Bites	1.7 %
Woolworths Gold	Cheese Straws	1.7 %
Arnott's	Vita-Weat 9 Grain Crispbread	1.8 %
Arnott's	Vita-Weat Cracked Pepper Crispbread	1.8 %
Arnott's	Vita-Weat Original Crispbread	1.8 %
Coles	Garlic Crackers	1.8 %
Damora	Sea Salt & Balsamic Vinegar Rice Cakes	1.8 %
Pureharvest	Organic Thin Linseed & Sesame Corn Cakes	1.8 %
Damora	Thin Rice & Corn Cakes	1.8 %
Roccas Deli	Garlic Baker Chips	1.8 %
SunRice	Seeds Rice & Grain Squares	1.8 %
Woolworths Gold	Cheese Bites	1.8 %
Woolworths Select	Garlic Crackers	1.8 %
Arnott's	Shapes Pizza	1.9 %
Arnott's	Vita-Weat Ancient Grains & Seeds Crispbread	1.9 %
Fantastic	Crisp'ns Salt & Balsamic Vinegar	1.9 %
Ricci's Bikkies	Olive Oil and Sea Salt Baked Pita Bread	1.9 %
SunRice	Salt & Balsamic Vinegar Thin Rice Cakes	1.9 %
Woolworths Select	Sesame & Cracked Pepper Wafer Crackers	1.9 %
Dick Smith's	Australian Water Cracker Biscuits	1.9 %
Arnott's	Jatz Cracked Pepper	2.0 %
Arnott's	Shapes Extreme BBQ Ribs	2.0 %

Brand	Label	% Sugar
Damora	Snackos Pizza	2.0 %
Stonebaker	Wholemeal with Olive Oil Artisan Baked Pita Bread	2.0 %
Vita Vigor	Organic Sesame Grissini Breadsticks	2.0 %
Woolworths Select	Original Wafer Crackers	2.0 %
Arnott's	Cruskits Rye	2.1 %
Arnott's	Poppy & Sesame Cracker	2.1 %
Arnott's	Savoy Cracked Pepper	2.1 %
Arnott's	Shapes Sensations Balsamic Vinegar & Sea Salt	2.1 %
Coles	Plain Rice Crackers	2.1 %
Simply Fine Food Company	Charcoal Lavoche Crispbread	2.1 %
Woolworths Homebrand	BBQ Flavoured Rice Crackers	2.1 %
Arnott's	Shapes Light & Crispy Tasty Cheddar & Chives	2.2 %
Arnott's	Shapes Sensations Roast Garlic & Parmesan	2.2 %
Coles	BBQ Snack Bites	2.2 %
Ricci's Bikkies	Pomodoro and Oregano Baked Pita Bread	2.2 %
Damora	Cheese Rice Crackers	2.2 %
Coles Simply Less	Crispbread	2.3 %
Orgran	Buckwheat Crispibread	2.3 %
Stonebaker	Tomato, Oregano & Parmesan Artisan Baked Pita Bread	2.3 %
Waterthins	Rice Fine Wafer Crackers	2.3 %
Woolworths Select	Sea Salt Crackers	2.3 %
Arnott's	Shapes Extreme Chilli	2.4 %

Brand	Label	% Sugar
Pureharvest	Organic Sesame Rice Cake Thins	2.4 %
Woolworths Select	Mediterranean Style Wafer Crackers	2.4 %
Arnott's	Shapes Sensations Basil Pesto & Parmesan	2.5 %
Arnott's	Vita-Weat Cheddar & Chives Rice Crackers	2.5 %
Coles	Original Wafer Crackers	2.5 %
Vita Vigor	Cheese Grissini Breadsticks	2.5 %
Waterthins	Natural Fine Wafer Crackers	2.5 %
Woolworths Select	Cracked Pepper Water Crackers	2.5 %
Coles	Pizza Snack Bites	2.6 %
Vita Vigor	Multigrain Grissini Breadsticks	2.6 %
Vita Vigor	Traditional Grissini Breadsticks	2.6 %
Damora	Barbecue Rice Crackers	2.6 %
Sakata	Barbecue Rice Crackers	2.6 %
Sakata	Classic Barbecue Rice Crackers	2.6 %
Arnott's	Shapes Light & Crispy Balsamic Vinegar & Sea Salt	2.7 %
OB Finest	Original Wafer Crackers	2.7 %
Vita Vigor	Garlic Grissini Breadsticks	2.7 %
Vita Vigor	Sesame Grissini Breadsticks	2.7 %
Damora	Pepper & Chives Fine Wafer Crackers	2.7 %
Finn Crisp	Original Rye Crispbread	2.7 %
Sakata	Roast Tomato & Balsamic Rice Crackers	2.7 %
SunRice	Roast Chicken Thin Rice Cakes	2.7 %
Woolworths Select	Snapz Cracked Pepper Crackers	2.7 %
Damora	Prista Original Crispbread	2.8 %

Brand	Label	% Sugar
Woolworths Select	Classic Water Crackers	2.8 %
Coles	Cracked Pepper Water Crackers	2.8 %
Nabisco	Premium Original Crispbread	2.8 %
Kurrajong Kitchen	Lavosh Thins Caramelized Onion & Sea Salt	2.9 %
Fantastic	Barbeque Rice Crackers	2.9 %
Kellogg's	Special K Cracker Crisps Sour Cream & Chives	2.9 %
Arnott's	Cheeseboard Crackers	3.0 %
Arnott's	Shapes Sensations Caramelised Onion & Cheddar	3.0 %
Arnott's	Shapes Sensations Honey Soy Chicken	3.0 %
Damora	Nice & Lite Rice Cracker Snacks	3.0 %
Damora	Sour Cream & Chives Rice Cakes	3.0 %
Ryvita	Crunch Dark Rye Crispbread	3.0 %
Sakata	Cheddar Cheese Rice Crackers	3.0 %
Sakata	Chicken Rice Crackers	3.0 %
Tucker's Natural	Four Cheese & Chives Gourmet Crackers	3.0 %

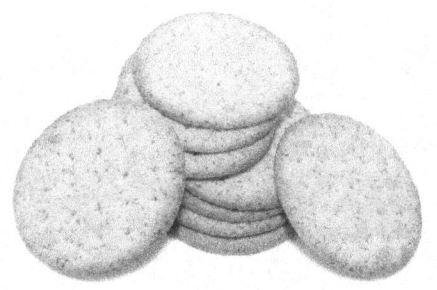

Biscuits - by brand

Brand	Label	% Sugar
Always Fresh	Wafer Crackers Roasted Sesame Crisp Bread	0.3 %
	Grissini Three Seed & Sea Salt Bread Sticks	0.8 %
	Crustini Olive Oil & Sea Salt Bruschetta Toasts	1.6 %
Arnott's	Original Cracked Pepper	0.1 %
	Sesame Water Crackers	0.1 %
	Supreme Crackers	0.1 %
	Cracked Pepper Water Crackers	0.2 %
	Salada Light Original	0.3 %
	Shapes Extreme Salt & Vinegar	0.3 %
	Salada Original	0.4 %
	Shapes Savoury	0.4 %
	Sao Crackers	0.5 %
	Vita-Weat Plain Rice Crackers	0.5 %
	Shapes Cheese & Bacon	0.6 %
	Vita-Weat Multigrain Rice Crackers	0.6 %
	Cruskits Corn	0.9 %
	Cruskits Rice	0.9 %
	Salada Multigrain	0.9 %
	Shapes BBQ	0.9 %
	Salada Wholemeal	1.1 %
	Cheds Crackers	1.2 %
	Savoy Original	1.3 %
	Sesame Wheat Crackers	1.3 %
	Shapes Extreme Peri Peri Chicken	1.4 %
	Shapes Nacho Cheese	1.4 %

Biscuits - by brand (continued)

Brand	Label	% Sugar
Arnott's	Shapes Cheddar	1.6 %
	Vita-Weat Sesame Crispbread	1.6 %
	Vita-Weat Five Super Seeds Crispbread	1.7 %
	Vita-Weat 9 Grain Crispbread	1.8 %
	Vita-Weat Cracked Pepper Crispbread	1.8 %
	Vita-Weat Original Crispbread	1.8 %
	Shapes Pizza	1.9 %
	Vita-Weat Ancient Grains & Seeds Crispbread	1.9 %
	Jatz Cracked Pepper	2.0 %
	Shapes Extreme BBQ Ribs	2.0 %
	Cruskits Rye	2.1 %
	Poppy & Sesame Cracker	2.1 %
	Savoy Cracked Pepper	2.1 %
	Shapes Sensations Balsamic Vinegar & Sea Salt	2.1 %
	Shapes Light & Crispy Tasty Cheddar & Chives	2.2 %
	Shapes Sensations Roast Garlic & Parmesan	2.2 %
	Shapes Extreme Chilli	2.4 %
	Shapes Sensations Basil Pesto & Parmesan	2.5 %
	Vita-Weat Cheddar & Chives Rice Crackers	2.5 %
	Shapes Light & Crispy Balsamic Vinegar & Sea Salt	2.7 %
	Cheeseboard Crackers	3.0 %
	Shapes Sensations Caramelised Onion & Cheddar	3.0 %
	Shapes Sensations Honey Soy Chicken	3.0 %
Belmont Biscuit Co.	Sugar Less Maria Biscuits	0.5 %

Brand	Label	% Sugar
Captain's Table	Classic Water Crackers	0.9 %
	Classic Water Crackers	0.9 %
	Cracked Pepper Water Crackers	0.9 %
	Cracked Pepper Water Crackers	0.9 %
	Sesame Seed Water Crackers	0.9 %
	Sesame Seed Water Crackers	0.9 %
Carr's	Garlic & Herbs Table Water Biscuits	1.5 %
	Sesame Seeds Table Water Biscuits	1.5 %
	Black Pepper Table Water Biscuits	1.6 %
	Table Water Biscuits	1.6 %
Coles	Brown Rice Crackers	0.7 %
	Seeds & Grains Brown Rice Crackers	0.8 %
	Thin Rice Cakes	0.9 %
	Garlic Crackers	1.8 %
	Plain Rice Crackers	2.1 %
	BBQ Snack Bites	2.2 %
	Original Wafer Crackers	2.5 %
	Pizza Snack Bites	2.6 %
	Cracked Pepper Water Crackers	2.8 %
Coles Simply Less	Crispbread	2.3 %
Damora	Plain Rice Crackers	0.2 %
	Brown Rice Crackers Original	0.5 %
	Mini Brown Rice Cakes Original	0.7 %
	Admiral's Quarters Cracked Pepper Water Crackers	0.9 %

Brand	Label	% Sugar
Damora	Admiral's Quarters Original Water Crackers	0.9 %
	Prista Lite Crispbread	0.9 %
	Brown Rice Crackers Multigrain	1.0 %
	Snackos Barbecue	1.0 %
	Original Thin Rice Cakes	1.1 %
	Snackos Cheese & Bacon	1.1 %
	Mini Brown Rice Cakes Chicken	1.5 %
	Vita Grain Sea Salt & Cracked Pepper Wholegrain Crackers	1.6 %
	Sanz Family Crackers	1.7 %
	Vita Grain Original Wholegrain Crackers	1.7 %
	Sea Salt & Balsamic Vinegar Rice Cakes	1.8 %
	Thin Rice & Corn Cakes	1.8 %
	Snackos Pizza	2.0 %
	Cheese Rice Crackers	2.2 %
	Barbecue Rice Crackers	2.6 %
	Pepper & Chives Fine Wafer Crackers	2.7 %
	Prista Original Crispbread	2.8 %
	Nice & Lite Rice Cracker Snacks	3.0 %
	Sour Cream & Chives Rice Cakes	3.0 %
Dick Smith's	Australian Water Cracker Biscuits	1.9 %
Eskal	Original Deli Crackers	1.4 %
Fantastic	Thinner Bite Sesame Black Rice Crackers	0.0 %
	Goodies Quinoa, Buckwheat, Millet & Amaranth Rice Crackers	1.1 %
	Salt & Vinegar Rice Crackers	1.3 %
Fantastic	Goodies 4 Grains Crackers	1.3 %

Brand	Label	% Sugar
Fantastic	Goodies Sesame, Poppy, Sunflower & Mustard Seeds Rice Crackers	1.5 %
	Crisp'ns Original	1.7 %
	Goodies 2 Seeds Crackers	1.7 %
	Crisp'ns Salt & Balsamic Vinegar	1.9 %
	Barbeque Rice Crackers	2.9 %
Fazer	Crisp Rye	1.4 %
Finn Crisp	Original Thin Rye Crispbread	1.6 %
	Original Rye Crispbread	2.7 %
Freelicious	Organic Amaranth & Protein Crispbread	1.4 %
Gullon	99.5 % Sugar Free Chocolate Chip Cookies	0.5 %
	99.5 % Sugar Free Digestive Biscuits	0.5 %
	99.5 % Sugar Free Shortbread Cookies	0.5 %
Kavli	Crispy Thin Crispbread	1.5 %
Kellogg's	Special K Cracker Crisps Sour Cream & Chives	2.9 %
Kurrajong Kitchen	Lavosh Thins Caramelized Onion & Sea Salt	2.9 %
Mary's Gone Crackers	Black Pepper Crackers	0.0 %
	Caraway Crackers	0.0 %
	Herb Crackers	0.0 %
	Jalapeno Crackers	0.0 %
	Onion Crackers	0.0 %
	Original Crackers	0.0 %
	Super Seed Crackers	0.0 %
Melinda's	Natural Crackers	0.3 %
Nabisco	Premium 98 % Fat Free Crispbread	0.9 %
	Premium Original Crispbread	2.8 %

Biscuits - by brand (continued)

Brand	Label	% Sugar
Naturally Good	Kasha Toasted Buckwheat Crispbread	1.3 %
OB Finest	Original Wafer Crackers	2.7 %
Orgran	Quinoa Wafer Crackers	0.5 %
	Essential Fibre Crispibread	0.6 %
	Chia Crispibread	0.7 %
	Chia Wafer Crackers	0.7 %
	Corn Crispibread	0.9 %
	Rice Crispibread	0.9 %
	Buckwheat Wafer Crackers	1.1 %
	Quinoa Crispibread	1.1 %
	Premium Multigrain Poppyseed Deli Crackers	1.5 %
	Buckwheat Crispibread	2.3 %
Peckish	BBQ Rice Snackers	0.9 %
	Brown Rice Crackers	0.9 %
	Brown Rice Crackers No Salt	0.9 %
	Cheddar Cheese Rice Crackers	0.9 %
	Cheese Rice Snackers	0.9 %
	Herb & Garlic Rice Crackers	0.9 %
	Original Rice Crackers	0.9 %
	Pizza Rice Snackers	0.9 %
	Pizza Supreme Rice Crackers	0.9 %
	Sea Salt & Vinegar Rice Crackers	0.9 %
	Sour Cream & Chive Rice Crackers	0.9 %
	Sour Cream & Chive Rice Snackers	0.9 %
	Sweet Chilli Rice Crackers	0.9 %
	Tangy BBQ Rice Crackers	0.9 %

Brand	Label	% Sugar
Pureharvest	Organic Thin Corn Cakes	0.2 %
	Organic Thin Quinoa Rice Cakes	0.4 %
	Organic Rice Cakes	0.5 %
	Organic Thin Linseed & Sesame Corn Cakes	1.8 %
	Organic Sesame Rice Cake Thins	2.4 %
Real Foods	Organic Sesame Corn Thins	0.4 %
	Original Corn Thins	0.4 %
	Multigrain Corn Thins	0.7 %
	Soy, Linseed & Chia Corn Thins	0.8 %
	Wholegrain Rice Thins	0.9 %
Red Tractor	Original Grain Oat Cakes	1.1 %
Ricci's Bikkies	Garlic, Olive & Parmesan Baked Pita Bread	1.5 %
	Herbed Baked Pita Bread	1.5 %
	Cheese & Chive Baked Pita Bread	1.7 %
	Olive Oil and Sea Salt Baked Pita Bread	1.9 %
	Pomodoro and Oregano Baked Pita Bread	2.2 %
Roccas Deli	Organic Fine Wafer Crackers	1.0 %
	Garlic Baker Chips	1.8 %
Ryvita	Crackerbread	1.5 %
	Crunch Dark Rye Crispbread	3.0 %
Sakata	Plain Rice Crackers	0.2 %
	Sea Salt & Cracked Pepper Rice Crackers	0.5 %
	Wholegrain Original Rice Crackers	1.7 %
	Barbecue Rice Crackers	2.6 %
	Classic Barbecue Rice Crackers	2.6 %

Biscuits - by brand (continued)

Brand	Label	% Sugar
Sakata	Roast Tomato & Balsamic Rice Crackers	2.7 %
	Cheddar Cheese Rice Crackers	3.0 %
	Chicken Rice Crackers	3.0 %
Simply Fine Food Company	Pepper Lavoche Crispbread	1.2 %
	Sesame & Poppy Lavoche Crispbread	1.2 %
	Parmesan Lavoche Crispbread	1.4 %
	Charcoal Lavoche Crispbread	2.1 %
Simply Wize	Cheese Deli Wafers	0.8 %
	Poppy Seed & Sea Salt Deli Wafers	0.8 %
Spiral Foods	Black Sesame Rice Crackers	0.5 %
	White Sesame Rice Crackers	0.5 %
	Tamari Rice Crackers	0.7 %
	Vegetable Rice Crackers	0.8 %
Stonebaker	Garlic, Olive, Rosemary & Parmesan Artisan Baked Pita Bread	1.3 %
	Wholemeal with Olive Oil Artisan Baked Pita Bread	2.0 %
	Tomato, Oregano & Parmesan Artisan Baked Pita Bread	2.3 %
SunRice	Original Thin Rice Cakes	0.8 %
	Wholegrain Brown Rice Original Mini Bites	0.8 %
	Original Thick Rice Cakes	0.9 %
SunRice	Quinoa Rice & Grain Squares	1.5 %
	Wholegrain Brown Rice Chicken Mini Bites	1.5 %
	Wild Rice Rice & Grain Squares	1.5 %
	Buckwheat Rice & Grain Squares	1.6 %

Brand	Label	% Sugar
SunRice	Linseed Rice & Grain Squares	1.6 %
	Wholegrain Brown Rice Salt & Vinegar Mini Bites	1.7 %
	Seeds Rice & Grain Squares	1.8 %
	Salt & Balsamic Vinegar Thin Rice Cakes	1.9 %
	Roast Chicken Thin Rice Cakes	2.7 %
Tucker's Natural	Four Cheese & Chives Gourmet Crackers	3.0 %
Valley Produce Company	Cracked Black Pepper Crackerthins	0.9 %
	Parmesan Cheese Crackerthins	0.9 %
Vita Vigor	Organic Sesame Grissini Breadsticks	2.0 %
	Cheese Grissini Breadsticks	2.5 %
	Multigrain Grissini Breadsticks	2.6 %
	Traditional Grissini Breadsticks	2.6 %
	Garlic Grissini Breadsticks	2.7 %
	Sesame Grissini Breadsticks	2.7 %
Walkers	Fine Oatcakes	0.5 %
	Thick & Crunchy Oatcakes	1.2 %
	Highland Oatcakes	1.6 %
Waterthins	Corn Fine Wafer Crackers	1.6 %
	Rice Fine Wafer Crackers	2.3 %
	Natural Fine Wafer Crackers	2.5 %
Woolworths Gold	Olive Oil Oatcakes	1.1 %
	Cheese & Seed Straws	1.4 %
	Cheese Palmiers	1.5 %

Brand	Label	% Sugar
Woolworths Gold	Cheese Pretzels	1.6 %
	Cheese Twists	1.6 %
	Cheese Straws	1.7 %
	Cheese Bites	1.8 %
Woolworths Homebrand	Plain Rice Crackers	0.0 %
	BBQ Flavoured Rice Crackers	2.1 %
Woolworths Macro Organic	Thick Rice Cakes	0.6 %
Woolworths Select	Sea Salt Brown Rice Crackers	0.3 %
	Original Thin Rice Cakes	0.6 %
	Multigrain Brown Rice Crackers	0.9 %
	Garlic Crackers	1.8 %
	Sesame & Cracked Pepper Wafer Crackers	1.9 %
	Original Wafer Crackers	2.0 %
	Sea Salt Crackers	2.3 %
	Mediterranean Style Wafer Crackers	2.4 %
	Cracked Pepper Water Crackers	2.5 %
	Snapz Cracked Pepper Crackers	2.7 %
	Classic Water Crackers	2.8 %

Ready Meals

If you don't have time to cook from scratch, there are some options that are low in sugar in the frozen Ready Meal section of the supermarket.

Many of these meals will contain seed oils. If you are concerned about this, then use the fat reckoner chart available at www.howmuchsugar.com to determine whether your choice is likely to be as low in seed oil as it is in sugar.

As always here is the list sorted by sugar content followed by the same list sorted by Brand.

Ready Meals - by sugar content

Brand	Label	% Sugar
Pitango	Solos Chicken & Mushroom Risotto	0.1 %
Lean Cuisine	Balanced Serve Lamb Koftas with Mildly Spiced Couscou	0.3 %
Latina Fresh	Beef Bolognese	0.4 %
Pitango	Chicken & Garlic Risotto	0.4 %
Woolworths	Created with Jamie Italian-Style Beef Meatballs	0.4 %
Woolworths	Salmon & Rice with Leek & Dill Cream Sauce	0.4 %
Woolworths	Slow Cooked Lamb Shanks with Rosemary Jus	0.4 %
Woolworths Select	Beef Madras with Rice	0.4 %
Woolworths Select	Butter Chicken with Rice	0.4 %
International Cuisine	Macaroni & Cheese	0.5 %
Latina Fresh	Chicken Risotto	0.5 %

Ready Meals - by sugar content (continued)

Brand	Label	% Sugar
On The Menu	3 Cheese Macaroni	0.5 %
The Good Meal Co.	Everyday Classics Beef Stroganoff & Rice	0.5 %
Woolworths	Beef Steak & Mushroom Sauce with Creamy Mashed Potato	0.5 %
Woolworths	Scalloped Potatoes with Bacon & Chives	0.5 %
CP Authentic Asia	King Prawn Wonton Soup with Noodles	0.6 %
On The Menu	Chicken Fettuccine	0.7 %
Woolworths	Creamy Boscaiola Penne	0.7 %
Coles Cuisine	Macaroni & Cheese	0.8 %
CP Authentic Asia	Red Thai Chicken Curry with Jasmine Rice	0.8 %
McCain	Fettucine Carbonara	0.8 %
SunRice	Global Kitchen Indian Style Spiced Rice with Chickpeas	0.8 %
The Element	Risotto with Roasted Butternut Pumpkin	0.8 %
Woolworths	Macaroni & Cheddar Cheese	0.8 %
Cucina Del Nonno	Gnocchi Napoli	0.9 %
International Cuisine	99 % Fat Free Beef in Red Wine Sauce with Mash	0.9 %
International Cuisine	99 % Fat Free Beef Stroganoff	0.9 %
The Element	Lasagna Chicken Mushroom Bolognese	0.9 %
Woolworths Select	Linguine Carbonara	0.9 %
Amy's Kitchen	Mexican Cheddar, Rice & Bean Burrito	1.0 %
Coles	Shepherd's Pie	1.0 %
Cucina Del Nonno	Lasagna Bolognese	1.0 %
Griff's	Lasagnette	1.0 %

Brand	Label	% Sugar
Latina Fresh	Chicken & Bacon Bake	1.0 %
McCain	Healthy Choice Slow Cooked Beef	1.0 %
McCain	Roast Beef	1.0 %
ME'N'U	Indian Lamb Rogan Josh with Potato & Basmati Rice	1.0 %
Street Food	Thai Chicken Curry Meal Pot	1.0 %
SunRice	Indian Chicken Korma Curry with Rice	1.0 %
Woolworths	Slow Cooked Lamb Shanks with Tomato & Barley Sauce4	1.0 %
Woolworths Select	Chicken & Mushroom Risotto	1.0 %
Andiamo Pasta Co.	Pesto Pasta Meal	1.1 %
Cucina Del Nonno	Roasted Beef Tortellini	1.1 %
Latina Fresh	Beef Stroganoff	1.1 %
Lean Cuisine	Balanced Serve Thai Green Chicken Curry with Rice	1.1 %
Lean Cuisine	Classic Chicken & Spinach Risotto	1.1 %
Pitango	Pumpkin, Leek & Spinach Risotto	1.1 %
Pitango	Solos Chicken & Herb Pasta Meal	1.1 %
Super Nature	Miso Salmon with Soba Noodles Super Foods	1.1 %
Woolworths Select	Beef Massaman Curry with Rice	1.1 %
Woolworths Select	Italian Classics Pumpkin & Parmesan Risotto	1.1 %
Clever Cooks	Homestyle Beef Lasagne	1.2 %
McCain	Roast Chicken	1.2 %
Pitango	Kids Salmon Risotto	1.2 %
Weight Watchers	Tuna Bake	1.2 %
Woolworths	Angus Bangers & Mash with Caramelised Onion Gravy	1.2 %

Brand	Label	% Sugar
Woolworths	Chicken Spiral Pasta Bake	1.2 %
Woolworths	Emily's Kitchen Beef Stroganoff with Rice	1.2 %
Amy's Kitchen	Light & Lean Pasta & Veggies	1.3 %
Coles	Satay Chicken	1.3 %
Lean Cuisine	Chinese Chicken and Sweet Corn Soup	1.3 %
Lean Cuisine	Steam Indian Chicken Tikka Masala	1.3 %
SunRice	Street Snack Mexican Chilli Con Carne with Rice	1.3 %
Woolworths Homebrand	Beef Lasagne	1.3 %
Woolworths Select	Chicken Korma with Rice	1.3 %
Coles	Macaroni Cheese	1.4 %
Griff's	Curried Prawns	1.4 %
Lean Cuisine	Malaysian Chicken Laksa Soup	1.4 %
Lean Cuisine	Steam Indian Beef Korma	1.4 %
Lean Cuisine	Steam Indian Style Butter Chicken with Rice	1.4 %
On The Menu	Roast Range Roast Chicken	1.4 %
Sunfresh	Noodle Pot Green Chicken Curry	1.4 %
The Good Meal Co.	Gluten Free Lentil & Veg Cottage Pie	1.4 %
Weight Watchers	Beef Hot Pot	1.4 %
Woolworths Select	Thai Green Chicken Curry with Rice	1.4 %
Woolworths Select	Yummy Meals Jungle Chicken Curry	1.4 %
CP Authentic Asia	Green Thai Chicken Curry with Jasmine Rice	1.5 %
International Cuisine	99 % Fat Free Chicken Risotto	1.5 %
Lean Cuisine	Classic Slow Cooked Beef Cannelloni	1.5 %

Ready Meals - by sugar content (continued)

Brand	Label	% Sugar
McCain	Healthy Choice Creamy Chicken Carbonara	1.5 %
On The Menu	Potato Bake	1.5 %
Pitango	Kids Macaroni Cheese	1.5 %
Pitango	Solos Macaroni Cheese with Bacon Pasta Meal	1.5 %
Pitango	Thai Green Chicken Curry	1.5 %
Ready Chef	Homestyle Cottage Pie	1.5 %
Woolworths Select	Beef Lasagne	1.5 %
Woolworths Select	Yummy Meals Sausages & Mashed Potato	1.5 %
Griff's	Pasta Carbonara	1.6 %
International Cuisine	Beef Lasagne	1.6 %
International Cuisine	Health & Vitality Satay Chicken	1.6 %
Lean Cuisine	Balanced Serve Chicken Florentine with Linguine	1.6 %
Lean Cuisine	Balanced Serve Satay Chicken Noodles	1.6 %
Lean Cuisine	Chinese Dumpling Soup	1.6 %
Lean Cuisine	Steam Slow Cook Beef	1.6 %
McCain	Healthy Choice Whole Grains Mexican Slow Cooked Beef	1.6 %
ME'N'U	Indian Butter Chicken with Basmati Rice	1.6 %
Pitango	Salmon, Dill & Pumpkin Risotto	1.6 %
The Good Meal Co.	Gluten Free Cottage Pie	1.6 %
Coles	Bechamel Beef Lasagne	1.7 %
Coles	Tuna Bake	1.7 %
Lean Cuisine	Balanced Serve Classic Beef Stroganoff with Pasta	1.7 %
Lean Cuisine	Steam Beef Penang Curry With Rice	1.7 %

Brand	Label	% Sugar
Lean Cuisine	Thai Dumpling Soup	1.7 %
McCain	Roast Lamb	1.7 %
Super Nature	Mediterranean Polenta Super Foods	1.7 %
The Good Meal Co.	Gluten Free Risotto Primavera	1.7 %
Weight Watchers	Beef Burgundy	1.7 %
Amy's Kitchen	Light & Lean 3 Cheese Penne Marinara	1.8 %
Coles	Thai Green Chicken Curry	1.8 %
Coles Cuisine	Shepherd's Pie	1.8 %
International Cuisine	Indian Style Butter Chicken	1.8 %
Lean Cuisine	Balanced Chicken and Chorizo Risotto	1.8 %
Lean Cuisine	Steam Meatball Arrabbiata	1.8 %
McCain	Healthy Choice Butter Chicken	1.8 %
McCain	Large Lasagne	1.8 %
ME'N'U	Italian Beef Lasagne	1.8 %
Super Nature	Thai Beef with Quinoa and Brown Rice Super Foods	1.8 %
Weight Watchers	Pumpkin & Ricotta Cannelloni	1.8 %
Woolworths Select	Beef Rogan Josh with Rice	1.8 %
Woolworths Select	Chicken Satay with Rice	1.8 %
Woolworths Select	Fresh Quiche Lorraine with Spring Onions	1.8 %
Amy's Kitchen	Gluten Free Broccoli & Cheddar Bake	1.9 %
Amy's Kitchen	Gluten Free Mexican Bean & Rice Burrito	1.9 %
Amy's Kitchen	Gluten Free Mexican Cheddar, Rice & Bean Burrito	1.9 %
Coles	Butter Chicken	1.9 %

Brand	Label	% Sugar
International Cuisine	99 % Fat Free Sundried Tomato, Chicken & Pasta	1.9 %
International Cuisine	Health & Vitality Chilli Con Carne	1.9 %
Latina Fresh	97 % Fat Free Lasagne with Angus Lean Beef & Vegetables	1.9 %
Lean Cuisine	Steam Satay Beef with Rice	1.9 %
McCain	Chicken Cacciatore	1.9 %
On The Menu	Chicken Parmigiana	1.9 %
On The Menu	Roast Range Roast Beef	1.9 %
On The Menu	Shepherd's Pie	1.9 %
Woolworths Select	Beef & Black Bean Sauce with Rice	1.9 %
Amy's Kitchen	Cheese Enchilada	2.0 %
Amy's Kitchen	Mexican Bean & Rice Burrito	2.0 %
Coles	Spaghetti Bolognese	2.0 %
International Cuisine	Health & Vitality Shepherd's Pie	2.0 %
Lean Cuisine	Steam Thai Red Chicken Curry with Rice	2.0 %
McCain	Chicken Parmigiana	2.0 %
McCain	Healthy Choice Chicken & Chorizo Paella	2.0 %
McCain	Healthy Choice Chinese Chicken & Cashews	2.0 %
McCain	Healthy Choice Honey Mustard Chicken	2.0 %
McCain	Healthy Choice Pasta Romana	2.0 %
Sara Lee	Gourmet Beef Lasagne	2.0 %
Sunfresh	Falafel & Lentil Tabouleh Salad Pot	2.0 %
SunRice	Thai Basil & Chilli Chicken Hokkien Noodles with Vegetables	2.0 %

Brand	Label	% Sugar
SunRice	Thai Red Chicken Curry with Jasmine Rice	2.0 %
Tutto Pasta	Lasagne Bolognese	2.0 %
Woolworths Select	Beef Reduced Fat Fresh Lasagne	2.0 %
Woolworths Select	Spinach & Ricotta Ravioli	2.0 %
Banquet	Fresh Beef Lasagne	2.1 %
International Cuisine	99 % Fat Free Mushroom Tortellini	2.1 %
International Cuisine	Health & Vitality Tuna Mornay	2.1 %
Latina Fresh	Spicy Chicken & Chorizo	2.1 %
Lean Cuisine	Balanced Serve Chicken & Vegetable Risotto	2.1 %
McCain	Beef & Bacon Pasta Bake	2.1 %
McCain	Tuna Mornay	2.1 %
Quick As Wok!	Chicken Laksa	2.1 %
Quick As Wok!	Red Chicken Curry	2.1 %
Sara Lee	Beef Lasagne	2.1 %
SunRice	Chinese Beef & Black Bean with Rice	2.1 %
SunRice	Indian Chicken Tikka Masala with Rice	2.1 %
The Good Meal Co.	Gluten Free Moroccan Tagine with Couscous	2.1 %
Weight Watchers	Chicken Parmigiana	2.1 %
Woolworths Select	Beef Fresh Lasagne	2.1 %
Amy's Kitchen	Mexican Tortilla Bake	2.2 %
Coles	Beef Madras Curry Pot	2.2 %
Lean Cuisine	Steam Cheese & Cracked Pepper Chicken with Pasta	2.2 %
McCain	Healthy Choice Whole Grains Malaysian Beef Curry	2.2 %

Ready Meals - by sugar content (continued)

Brand	Label	% Sugar
McCain	Healthy Choice Whole Grains Thai Beef & Basil Stir Fry	2.2 %
McCain	Lasagne	2.2 %
ME'N'U	Single Serve 3 Cheese Cannelloni	2.2 %
On The Menu	Cottage Pie	2.2 %
The Element	Cannelloni Ricotta Spinach	2.2 %
Tutto Pasta	Vegetarian Lasagne	2.2 %
Weight Watchers	Chicken Tikka Masala	2.2 %
Woolworths Select	Fresh Pasta Bake Penne & Bolognese	2.2 %
Woolworths Select	Fresh Pasta Bake Spaghetti & Meatballs	2.2 %
Coles Smart Buy	Beef Lasagne	2.3 %
Cucina Del Nonno	Lasagna Vegetarian	2.3 %
On The Menu	Pub Favourites Chicken Kiev	2.3 %
Quick As Wok!	Singapore Noodles	2.3 %
SunRice	Thai Green Chicken Curry with Jasmine Rice	2.3 %
The Good Meal Co.	Everyday Classics Cottage Pie	2.3 %
Weight Watchers	Beef & Tomato Bolognese	2.3 %
Weight Watchers	Roasted Sweet Potato & Pumpkin Risotto	2.3 %
Weight Watchers	Thai Chicken Curry	2.3 %
Woolworths	Classic Spaghetti Bolognese	2.3 %
Woolworths	Corned Beef & Mustard Sauce with Creamy Mash & Red Cabbage	2.3 %
Amy's Kitchen	Gluten Free Rice Mac & Cheese	2.4 %
b.e. Ready Meals	Mini Beef Burritos	2.4 %
Banquet	Fresh Quiche Lorraine	2.4 %
Coles	Thai Red Chicken Curry	2.4 %

Brand	Label	% Sugar
Latina Fresh	Italian Meatballs	2.4 %
Lean Cuisine	Steam Atlantic Salmon with Pasta	2.4 %
McCain	Shepherd's Pie	2.4 %
On The Menu	Moroccan Meatballs	2.4 %
On The Menu	Spaghetti & Meatballs	2.4 %
Pitango	Vegetable Korma Curry	2.4 %
Super Nature	Chicken, Asparagus and Pearl Barley Risotto Super Foods	2.4 %
The Element	Risotto with Assorted Mushrooms	2.4 %
McCain	Healthy Choice Beef Lasagne	2.5 %
McCain	Spaghetti Bolognese	2.5 %
Pitango	Butter Chicken Curry	2.5 %
Pitango	Kids Spaghetti Bolognese	2.5 %
Ready Chef	Homestyle Beef Lasagne	2.5 %
Sunfresh	Down to Earth Roasted Vegetable Warm Salad	2.5 %
Sunfresh	Pesto Risoni & Feta Salad Pot	2.5 %
SunRice	Coconut Chicken Rice Noodles with Vegetables	2.5 %
The Good Meal Co.	Gluten Free Butter Chickpea & Veg Curry	2.5 %
Woolworths	Chicken Korma with Basmati Rice	2.5 %
Woolworths Select	Family Sized Beef Lasagne	2.5 %
Woolworths Select	Fresh Quiche Pumpkin & Capsicum with Parmesan	2.5 %
Woolworths Select	Spaghetti Bolognese	2.5 %
Amy's Kitchen	Light & Lean Spaghetti Italiano	2.6 %
Coles	Lamb Rogan Josh Curry Pot	2.6 %

Ready Meals - by sugar content (continued)

Brand	Label	% Sugar
Griff's	Pasta Bolognese	2.6 %
Lean Cuisine	Balanced Serve Honey Soy Beef with Wholemeal Noodles	2.6 %
Lean Cuisine	Classic Chilli Con Carne with Rice	2.6 %
Super Nature	Split Pea and Lentil Dhal Super Foods	2.6 %
Weight Watchers	Creamy Mushroom & Pumpkin Risotto	2.6 %
Woolworths	Angus Beef Lasagne	2.6 %
Woolworths	Ricotta & Spinach Cannelloni	2.6 %
Andiamo Pasta Co.	Tomato, Onion & Herbs Pasta Meal	2.7 %
Hedy's	Leek & Bacon Quiche	2.7 %
Lean Cuisine	Balanced Serve Spaghetti Bolognese	2.7 %
McCain	Healthy Choice Basil Pesto Chicken	2.7 %
McCain	Healthy Choice Thai Red Curry	2.7 %
Tutto Pasta	Spinach & Ricotta Cannelloni	2.7 %
Weight Watchers	Chicken Risotto	2.7 %
Weight Watchers	Satay Style Chicken	2.7 %
Woolworths	Lamb Rogan Josh with Basmati Rice	2.7 %
Black & Gold	Beef Lasagne	2.8 %
Hedy's	Quiche Lorraine	2.8 %
International Cuisine	Health & Vitality Basil Chicken	2.8 %
Latina Fresh	Lasagne with Angus Beef & Hearty Vegetables	2.8 %
Lean Cuisine	Balanced Serve Creamy Chicken & Basil with Spaghetti	2.8 %
Lean Cuisine	Balanced Serve Creamy Salmon & Dill Pasta	2.8 %
Lucha Libre	Beef Burrito with Corn Esquites	2.8 %

Ready Meals - by sugar content (continued)

Brand	Label	% Sugar
ME'N'U	Homestyle Quiche Lorraine	2.8 %
On The Menu	Beef Lasagne	2.8 %
The Good Meal Co.	Gluten Free Creamy Tomato Fusilli with Chicken & Bacon	2.8 %
Weight Watchers	Spaghetti & Meatballs	2.8 %
Amy's Kitchen	Vegetable Lasagne	2.9 %
Andiamo Pasta Co.	Tomato, Garlic & Basil Pasta Meal	2.9 %
Coles	Honey Mustard Chicken	2.9 %
Coles	Sweet & Sour Chicken	2.9 %
International Cuisine	99 % Fat Free Vegetable Cannelloni	2.9 %
Lean Cuisine	Steam Tortellini with Beef & Parmesan in Creamy Sundried Tomato Sauce	2.9 %
McCain	Healthy Choice Whole Grains Italian Beef & Chia Meatballs	2.9 %
SunRice	Indian Butter Chicken Curry with Rice	2.9 %
Woolworths	Flip n Go Pasta Salad with Tomato Pesto and Bocconcini	2.9 %
Amy's Kitchen	Margherita Pizza	3.0 %
McCain	Healthy Choice Beef Florentine	3.0 %
Pitango	Kids Very Mild Chicken Curry	3.0 %
Pitango	Tomato, Feta & Basil Risotto	3.0 %
Quick As Wok!	Chicken Chow Mein	3.0 %
Sunfresh	Chicken & Quinoa Salad Pot	3.0 %
SunRice	Beef & Oyster Sauce Hokkien Noodles with Vegetables	3.0 %
Weight Watchers	Country Chicken Casserole	3.0 %
Woolworths	Butter Chicken with Basmati Rice	3.0 %
Woolworths Select	Yummy Meals Spaghetti & Meatballs	3.0 %

Ready Meals - by brand

Brand	Label	% Sugar
Amy's Kitchen	Mexican Cheddar, Rice & Bean Burrito	1.0 %
	Light & Lean Pasta & Veggies	1.3 %
	Light & Lean 3 Cheese Penne Marinara	1.8 %
	Gluten Free Broccoli & Cheddar Bake	1.9 %
	Gluten Free Mexican Bean & Rice Burrito	1.9 %
	Gluten Free Mexican Cheddar, Rice & Bean Burrito	1.9 %
	Cheese Enchilada	2.0 %
	Mexican Bean & Rice Burrito	2.0 %
	Mexican Tortilla Bake	2.2 %
	Gluten Free Rice Mac & Cheese	2.4 %
	Light & Lean Spaghetti Italiano	2.6 %
	Vegetable Lasagne	2.9 %
	Margherita Pizza	3.0 %
Andiamo Pasta Co.	Pesto Pasta Meal	1.1 %
	Tomato, Onion & Herbs Pasta Meal	2.7 %
	Tomato, Garlic & Basil Pasta Meal	2.9 %
b.e. Ready Meals	Mini Beef Burritos	2.4 %
Banquet	Fresh Beef Lasagne	2.1 %
	Fresh Quiche Lorraine	2.4 %
Black & Gold	Beef Lasagne	2.8 %
Clever Cooks	Homestyle Beef Lasagne	1.2 %
Coles	Shepherd's Pie	1.0 %
	Satay Chicken	1.3 %
	Macaroni Cheese	1.4 %

Brand	Label	% Sugar
Coles	Bechamel Beef Lasagne	1.7 %
	Tuna Bake	1.7 %
	Thai Green Chicken Curry	1.8 %
	Butter Chicken	1.9 %
	Spaghetti Bolognese	2.0 %
	Beef Madras Curry Pot	2.2 %
	Thai Red Chicken Curry	2.4 %
	Lamb Rogan Josh Curry Pot	2.6 %
	Honey Mustard Chicken	2.9 %
	Sweet & Sour Chicken	2.9 %
Coles Cuisine	Macaroni & Cheese	0.8 %
	Shepherd's Pie	1.8 %
Coles Smart Buy	Beef Lasagne	2.3 %
CP Authentic Asia	King Prawn Wonton Soup with Noodles	0.6 %
	Red Thai Chicken Curry with Jasmine Rice	0.8 %
	Green Thai Chicken Curry with Jasmine Rice	1.5 %
Cucina Del Nonno	Gnocchi Napoli	0.9 %
	Lasagna Bolognese	1.0 %
	Roasted Beef Tortellini	1.1 %
	Lasagna Vegetarian	2.3 %
Griff's	Lasagnette	1.0 %
	Curried Prawns	1.4 %
	Pasta Carbonara	1.6 %
Griff's	Pasta Bolognese	2.6 %

Brand	Label	% Sugar
Hedy's	Leek & Bacon Quiche	2.7 %
	Quiche Lorraine	2.8 %
International Cuisine	Macaroni & Cheese	0.5 %
	99 % Fat Free Beef in Red Wine Sauce with Mash	0.9 %
	99 % Fat Free Beef Stroganoff	0.9 %
	99 % Fat Free Chicken Risotto	1.5 %
	Beef Lasagne	1.6 %
	Health & Vitality Satay Chicken	1.6 %
	Indian Style Butter Chicken	1.8 %
	99 % Fat Free Sundried Tomato, Chicken & Pasta	1.9 %
	Health & Vitality Chilli Con Carne	1.9 %
	Health & Vitality Shepherd's Pie	2.0 %
	99 % Fat Free Mushroom Tortellini	2.1 %
	Health & Vitality Tuna Mornay	2.1 %
	Health & Vitality Basil Chicken	2.8 %
	99 % Fat Free Vegetable Cannelloni	2.9 %
Latina Fresh	Beef Bolognese	0.4 %
	Chicken Risotto	0.5 %
	Chicken & Bacon Bake	1.0 %
	Beef Stroganoff	1.1 %
	97 % Fat Free Lasagne with Angus Lean Beef & Vegetables	1.9 %
	Spicy Chicken & Chorizo	2.1 %
Latina Fresh	Italian Meatballs	2.4 %

Brand	Label	% Sugar
Latina Fresh	Lasagne with Angus Beef & Hearty Vegetables	2.8 %
Lean Cuisine	Balanced Serve Lamb Koftas with Mildly Spiced Couscou	0.3 %
	Balanced Serve Thai Green Chicken Curry with Rice	1.1 %
	Classic Chicken & Spinach Risotto	1.1 %
	Chinese Chicken and Sweet Corn Soup	1.3 %
	Steam Indian Chicken Tikka Masala	1.3 %
	Malaysian Chicken Laksa Soup	1.4 %
	Steam Indian Beef Korma	1.4 %
	Steam Indian Style Butter Chicken with Rice	1.4 %
	Classic Slow Cooked Beef Cannelloni	1.5 %
	Balanced Serve Chicken Florentine with Linguine	1.6 %
	Balanced Serve Satay Chicken Noodles	1.6 %
	Chinese Dumpling Soup	1.6 %
	Steam Slow Cook Beef	1.6 %
	Balanced Serve Classic Beef Stroganoff with Pasta	1.7 %
	Steam Beef Penang Curry With Rice	1.7 %
	Thai Dumpling Soup	1.7 %
	Balanced Chicken and Chorizo Risotto	1.8 %
	Steam Meatball Arrabbiata	1.8 %
	Steam Satay Beef with Rice	1.9 %
	Steam Thai Red Chicken Curry with Rice	2.0 %
Lean Cuisine	Balanced Serve Chicken & Vegetable Risotto	2.1 %

Ready Meals - by brand (continued)

Brand	Label	% Sugar
Lean Cuisine	Steam Cheese & Cracked Pepper Chicken with Pasta	2.2 %
	Steam Atlantic Salmon with Pasta	2.4 %
	Balanced Serve Honey Soy Beef with Wholemeal Noodles	2.6 %
	Classic Chilli Con Carne with Rice	2.6 %
	Balanced Serve Spaghetti Bolognese	2.7 %
	Balanced Serve Creamy Chicken & Basil with Spaghetti	2.8 %
	Balanced Serve Creamy Salmon & Dill Pasta	2.8 %
	Steam Tortellini with Beef & Parmesan in Creamy Sundried Tomato Sauce	2.9 %
Lucha Libre	Beef Burrito with Corn Esquites	2.8 %
McCain	Fettucine Carbonara	0.8 %
	Healthy Choice Slow Cooked Beef	1.0 %
	Roast Beef	1.0 %
	Roast Chicken	1.2 %
	Healthy Choice Creamy Chicken Carbonara	1.5 %
	Healthy Choice Whole Grains Mexican Slow Cooked Beef	1.6 %
	Roast Lamb	1.7 %
	Healthy Choice Butter Chicken	1.8 %
	Large Lasagne	1.8 %
	Chicken Cacciatore	1.9 %
	Chicken Parmigiana	2.0 %
	Healthy Choice Chicken & Chorizo Paella	2.0 %
McCain	Healthy Choice Chinese Chicken & Cashews	2.0 %

Brand	Label	% Sugar
McCain	Healthy Choice Honey Mustard Chicken	2.0 %
	Healthy Choice Pasta Romana	2.0 %
	Beef & Bacon Pasta Bake	2.1 %
	Tuna Mornay	2.1 %
	Healthy Choice Whole Grains Malaysian Beef Curry	2.2 %
	Healthy Choice Whole Grains Thai Beef & Basil Stir Fry	2.2 %
	Lasagne	2.2 %
	Shepherd's Pie	2.4 %
	Healthy Choice Beef Lasagne	2.5 %
	Spaghetti Bolognese	2.5 %
	Healthy Choice Basil Pesto Chicken	2.7 %
	Healthy Choice Thai Red Curry	2.7 %
	Healthy Choice Whole Grains Italian Beef & Chia Meatballs	2.9 %
	Healthy Choice Beef Florentine	3.0 %
ME'N'U	Indian Lamb Rogan Josh with Potato & Basmati Rice	1.0 %
	Indian Butter Chicken with Basmati Rice	1.6 %
	Italian Beef Lasagne	1.8 %
	Single Serve 3 Cheese Cannelloni	2.2 %
	Homestyle Quiche Lorraine	2.8 %
On The Menu	3 Cheese Macaroni	0.5 %
	Chicken Fettuccine	0.7 %
On The Menu	Roast Range Roast Chicken	1.4 %
	Potato Bake	1.5 %

Brand	Label	% Sugar
On The Menu	Chicken Parmigiana	1.9 %
	Roast Range Roast Beef	1.9 %
	Shepherd's Pie	1.9 %
	Cottage Pie	2.2 %
	Pub Favourites Chicken Kiev	2.3 %
	Moroccan Meatballs	2.4 %
	Spaghetti & Meatballs	2.4 %
	Beef Lasagne	2.8 %
Pitango	Solos Chicken & Mushroom Risotto	0.1 %
	Chicken & Garlic Risotto	0.4 %
	Pumpkin, Leek & Spinach Risotto	1.1 %
	Solos Chicken & Herb Pasta Meal	1.1 %
	Kids Salmon Risotto	1.2 %
	Kids Macaroni Cheese	1.5 %
	Solos Macaroni Cheese with Bacon Pasta Meal	1.5 %
	Thai Green Chicken Curry	1.5 %
	Salmon, Dill & Pumpkin Risotto	1.6 %
	Vegetable Korma Curry	2.4 %
	Butter Chicken Curry	2.5 %
	Kids Spaghetti Bolognese	2.5 %
	Kids Very Mild Chicken Curry	3.0 %
	Tomato, Feta & Basil Risotto	3.0 %
Quick As Wok!	Chicken Laksa	2.1 %
	Red Chicken Curry	2.1 %

Brand	Label	% Sugar
Quick As Wok!	Singapore Noodles	2.3 %
	Chicken Chow Mein	3.0 %
Ready Chef	Homestyle Cottage Pie	1.5 %
	Homestyle Beef Lasagne	2.5 %
Sara Lee	Gourmet Beef Lasagne	2.0 %
	Beef Lasagne	2.1 %
Street Food	Thai Chicken Curry Meal Pot	1.0 %
Sunfresh	Noodle Pot Green Chicken Curry	1.4 %
	Falafel & Lentil Tabouleh Salad Pot	2.0 %
	Down to Earth Roasted Vegetable Warm Salad	2.5 %
	Pesto Risoni & Feta Salad Pot	2.5 %
	Chicken & Quinoa Salad Pot	3.0 %
SunRice	Global Kitchen Indian Style Spiced Rice with Chickpeas	0.8 %
	Indian Chicken Korma Curry with Rice	1.0 %
	Street Snack Mexican Chilli Con Carne with Rice	1.3 %
	Thai Basil & Chilli Chicken Hokkien Noodles with Vegetables	2.0 %
	Thai Red Chicken Curry with Jasmine Rice	2.0 %
	Chinese Beef & Black Bean with Rice	2.1 %
	Indian Chicken Tikka Masala with Rice	2.1 %
	Thai Green Chicken Curry with Jasmine Rice	2.3 %
SunRice	Coconut Chicken Rice Noodles with Vegetables	2.5 %
	Indian Butter Chicken Curry with Rice	2.9 %

Brand	Label	% Sugar
SunRice	Beef & Oyster Sauce Hokkien Noodles with Vegetables	3.0 %
Super Nature	Miso Salmon with Soba Noodles Super Foods	1.1 %
	Mediterranean Polenta Super Foods	1.7 %
	Thai Beef with Quinoa and Brown Rice Super Foods	1.8 %
	Chicken, Asparagus and Pearl Barley Risotto Super Foods	2.4 %
	Split Pea and Lentil Dhal Super Foods	2.6 %
The Element	Risotto with Roasted Butternut Pumpkin	0.8 %
	Lasagna Chicken Mushroom Bolognese	0.9 %
	Cannelloni Ricotta Spinach	2.2 %
	Risotto with Assorted Mushrooms	2.4 %
The Good Meal Co.	Everyday Classics Beef Stroganoff & Rice	0.5 %
	Gluten Free Lentil & Veg Cottage Pie	1.4 %
	Gluten Free Cottage Pie	1.6 %
	Gluten Free Risotto Primavera	1.7 %
	Gluten Free Moroccan Tagine with Couscous	2.1 %
	Everyday Classics Cottage Pie	2.3 %
	Gluten Free Butter Chickpea & Veg Curry	2.5 %
	Gluten Free Creamy Tomato Fusilli with Chicken & Bacon	2.8 %
Tutto Pasta	Lasagne Bolognese	2.0 %
Tutto Pasta	Vegetarian Lasagne	2.2 %
	Spinach & Ricotta Cannelloni	2.7 %
Weight Watchers	Tuna Bake	1.2 %

Ready Meals - by brand (continued)

Brand	Label	% Sugar
Weight Watchers	Beef Hot Pot	1.4 %
	Beef Burgundy	1.7 %
	Pumpkin & Ricotta Cannelloni	1.8 %
	Chicken Parmigiana	2.1 %
	Chicken Tikka Masala	2.2 %
	Beef & Tomato Bolognese	2.3 %
	Roasted Sweet Potato & Pumpkin Risotto	2.3 %
	Thai Chicken Curry	2.3 %
	Creamy Mushroom & Pumpkin Risotto	2.6 %
	Chicken Risotto	2.7 %
	Satay Style Chicken	2.7 %
	Spaghetti & Meatballs	2.8 %
	Country Chicken Casserole	3.0 %
Woolworths	Created with Jamie Italian-Style Beef Meatballs	0.4 %
	Salmon & Rice with Leek & Dill Cream Sauce	0.4 %
	Slow Cooked Lamb Shanks with Rosemary Jus	0.4 %
	Beef Steak & Mushroom Sauce with Creamy Mashed Potato	0.5 %
	Scalloped Potatoes with Bacon & Chives	0.5 %
	Creamy Boscaiola Penne	0.7 %
	Macaroni & Cheddar Cheese	0.8 %
Woolworths	Slow Cooked Lamb Shanks with Tomato & Barley Sauce4	1.0 %
	Angus Bangers & Mash with Caramelised Onion Gravy	1.2 %

Ready Meals - by brand (continued)

Brand	Label	% Sugar
Woolworths	Chicken Spiral Pasta Bake	1.2 %
	Emily's Kitchen Beef Stroganoff with Rice	1.2 %
	Classic Spaghetti Bolognese	2.3 %
	Corned Beef & Mustard Sauce with Creamy Mash & Red Cabbage	2.3 %
	Chicken Korma with Basmati Rice	2.5 %
	Angus Beef Lasagne	2.6 %
	Ricotta & Spinach Cannelloni	2.6 %
	Lamb Rogan Josh with Basmati Rice	2.7 %
	Flip n Go Pasta Salad with Tomato Pesto and Bocconcini	2.9 %
	Butter Chicken with Basmati Rice	3.0 %
Woolworths Homebrand	Beef Lasagne	1.3 %
Woolworths Select	Beef Madras with Rice	0.4 %
	Butter Chicken with Rice	0.4 %
	Linguine Carbonara	0.9 %
	Chicken & Mushroom Risotto	1.0 %
	Beef Massaman Curry with Rice	1.1 %
	Italian Classics Pumpkin & Parmesan Risotto	1.1 %
	Chicken Korma with Rice	1.3 %
Woolworths Select	Thai Green Chicken Curry with Rice	1.4 %
	Yummy Meals Jungle Chicken Curry	1.4 %
	Beef Lasagne	1.5 %

Brand	Label	% Sugar
Woolworths Select	Yummy Meals Sausages & Mashed Potato	1.5 %
	Beef Rogan Josh with Rice	1.8 %
	Chicken Satay with Rice	1.8 %
	Fresh Quiche Lorraine with Spring Onions	1.8 %
	Beef & Black Bean Sauce with Rice	1.9 %
	Beef Reduced Fat Fresh Lasagne	2.0 %
	Spinach & Ricotta Ravioli	2.0 %
	Beef Fresh Lasagne	2.1 %
	Fresh Pasta Bake Penne & Bolognese	2.2 %
	Fresh Pasta Bake Spaghetti & Meatballs	2.2 %
	Family Sized Beef Lasagne	2.5 %
	Fresh Quiche Pumpkin & Capsicum with Parmesan	2.5 %
	Spaghetti Bolognese	2.5 %
	Yummy Meals Spaghetti & Meatballs	3.0 %

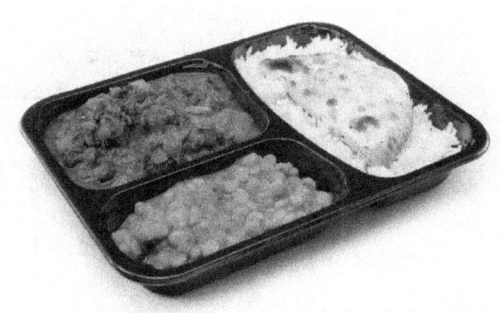

Frozen Pizza

Sometimes even a ready meal is just too much bother. If you just want a pizza you can shove from freezer to oven, there are (believe it or not) some options in your local supermarket. Here they are. Once again many of these pizza's will contain seed oils. If you are concerned about this, then use the fat reckoner chart available at www.howmuchsugar.com to determine whether your choice is likely to be as low in seed oil as it is in sugar.

Brand	Label	% Sugar
Woolworths Gold	Calabrese Salami & Mozzarella Pizza	0.8 %
Woolworths Gold	Free Range Chicken & Pancetta Pizza	0.9 %
Woolworths Gold	Margherita with Basil Infused Oil Pizza	1.2 %
Dr. Oetker	Ristorante Funghi Pizza	1.6 %
Dr. Oetker	Papa Giuseppi's Mediterranean Panini	1.8 %
Dr. Oetker	Papa Giuseppi's Tomato & Cheese Panini	1.8 %
Dr. Oetker	Ristorante Spinaci Pizza	1.8 %
Dr. Oetker	Ristorante Mozzarella Pizza	2.0 %
Dr. Oetker	Ristorante Quattro Formaggi Pizza	2.0 %
Woolworths Select	Mushroom & Mozzarella Pizza	2.0 %
Dr. Oetker	Papa Giuseppi's Pepperoni Bakehouse Crust Pizza	2.1 %
Dr. Oetker	Papa Giuseppi's Roast Pumpkin, Feta & Spinach Bakehouse Crust Pizza	2.2 %
Cucina Del Nonno	Calabrese Pizza	2.3 %
Della Rosa	Spicy Italian Gourmet Pizza	2.3 %
Della Rosa	Char Grilled Chicken Gourmet Pizza	2.5 %
Woolworths Select	Quattro Formaggi Pizza	2.5 %

Fast Food

Supermarkets aren't the only place you'll be buying food prepared by others. To cover off the majority of the market for 'restaurant' food, in this section, I've analysed the menu's of the major fast food chains.

> **WARNING: All fried food sold in these restaurants in Australia has been fried in seed oils and should be avoided if you are concerned about seed oils.**

Subway Restaurants

Category	Item	% Sugar
Sandwiches with 6g of Fat or Less	Chicken Strips	2.3 %
	Ham	3.0 %
	Oven Roasted Chicken	2.4 %
	Turkey	2.8 %
	Turkey & Ham	2.8 %
	Subway Club	3.0 %
Sandwiches	Chicken & Bacon Ranch Melt	2.0 %
	Chicken Classic	2.7 %
	Chicken Parmigiana	2.6 %
	Chicken Schnitzel	2.4 %
	Italian B.M.T.	2.8 %
	Steak & Cheese	2.3 %
	Subway Melt	2.5 %

Subway Restaurants (continued)

Category	Item	% Sugar
Sandwiches	Tuna	2.3 %
Flatbread Sandwiches	Chicken Strips	1.5 %
	Ham	2.1 %
	Roast Beef	2.6 %
	Oven Roasted Chicken	1.7 %
	Turkey	1.8 %
	Turkey & Ham	1.9 %
	Subway Club	2.1 %
	Veggie Delite	2.1 %
Mini Subs	Chicken Strips	2.0 %
	Turkey	2.7 %
Salads with 6g of Fat or Less	Chicken Strips	1.4 %
	Chicken Teriyaki	2.8 %
	Ham	1.8 %
	Oven Roasted Chicken	1.5 %
	Roast Beef	2.1 %
	Turkey	1.6 %
	Turkey & Ham	1.7 %
	Subway Club	1.8 %
	Veggie Delite	1.7 %
Wraps	Chicken Strips	1.9 %
	Ham	2.1 %
	Roast Beef	2.6 %
	Turkey	1.8 %
	Turkey & Ham	1.9 %

Subway Restaurants (continued)

Category	Item	% Sugar
Wraps	Subway Club	2.1 %
	Veggie Delite	2.1 %
Breakfast Sandwiches	Shortcut Bacon, Poached Egg & Cheese	2.5 %
	Poached Egg & Cheese	2.8 %
	Ham, Poached Egg & Cheese	2.8 %
Flatbread Breakfast Sandwiches	Shortcut Bacon, Poached Egg & Cheese	1.6 %
	Poached Egg & Cheese	1.8 %
	Ham, Poached Egg & Cheese	1.9 %
Breads	6-Inch Flatbread	2.1 %
	Wrap	2.0 %
Toppings	Mayonnaise	0.0 %
	Ranch Dressing	1.0 %
Cheese	Cheddar Cheese	1.7 %
	Mozzarella Cheese	0.5 %
	Old English Cheese	1.1 %
	Swiss Cheese	0.0 %
Vegetables	Capsicum	2.4 %
	Cucumbers	1.7 %
	Lettuce	0.7 %
	Pickles	0.0 %
	Olives	0.9 %
	Spinach	0.4 %
	Tomatoes	2.6 %

McDonald's

Category	Item	% Sugar
Create Your Taste	Chipotle Burger	1.7 %
Beef	Big Mac	2.9 %
	Grand Angus	2.0 %
	McFeast	2.9 %
	Mighty Angus	2.9 %
	Double Quarter Pounder	2.3 %
	Steak Roll	1.5 %
Chicken and Fish	Chicken Nuggets	0.5 %
	Chicken Mc Bites	0.6 %
	Chicken & Cheese	1.9 %
	Chicken & Mayo	2.0 %
	Crispy Chicken Deluxe	2.1 %
	Grilled Chicken Deluxe	2.4 %
	South West Crispy Chicken Burger	2.4 %
	South West Grilled Chicken Burger	2.7 %
	Spicy Jalapeno Grilled Chicken Burger	2.7 %
	McChicken	1.7 %
	Filet-o-Fish	2.0 %
Wraps	Crispy Chicken Snack Wrap	1.6 %
	Grilled Chicken Snack Wrap	2.0 %
	Chicken & Aioli McWrap - Crispy Chicken	1.8 %
	Chicken & Aioli McWrap - Grilled Chicken	2.1 %
	Chicken & Spicy Mayo McWrap - Crispy Chicken	1.9 %

McDonald's (continued)

Category	Item	% Sugar
Wraps	Chicken & Spicy Mayo McWrap - Grilled Chicken	2.2 %
	Steak and Aioli McWrap	2.2 %
French Fries	French Fries	0.4 %
Salads	Warm Chicken Salad - Crispy Chicken	1.9 %
	Warm Chicken Salad - Grilled Chicken	2.1 %
	Crunchy Noodle Salad - Crispy Chicken	1.8 %
	Crunchy Noodle Salad - Grilled Chicken	2.0 %
	Steak Salad	2.2 %
	Garden Salad	1.1 %
Breakfast	Deluxe Brekkie Roll	2.0 %
	Hash Brown	0.4 %
	Ham & Cheese Pocket	2.0 %
	McMuffin - Bacon & Egg	1.6 %
	McMuffin - BLT	2.0 %
	McMuffin - Plain	2.0 %
	McMuffin - Sausage	1.6 %
	McMuffin - Sausage and Egg	1.2 %
	Steak & Egg Wrap	3.0 %
McCafe	Veggie Omelette and Ham Sandwich	2.7 %
	Sausage Omelette and Chorizo Sandwich	1.6 %
	Croissant with Ham & Cheese	2.0 %
	Cheesy Chorizo Roll	2.4 %

McDonald's (continued)

Category	Item	% Sugar
McCafe	Cheese & Tomato Toasted Sandwiches	2.4 %
	Cheese & Tomato Toasted Sandwiches	2.0 %
	Ham & Cheese Toasted Sandwiches	2.1 %
	Ham & Cheese Toasted Sandwiches	1.8 %
	Ham, Cheese & Tomato Toasted Sandwiches	2.1 %
	Ham, Cheese & Tomato Toasted Sandwiches	1.8 %
	Ruben Sandwich	2.0 %
	Roast Beef & Cheddar Sandwich	1.7 %
	Chicken Pesto Sandwich	2.5 %
	Chorizo & Cheese Frittata	2.0 %

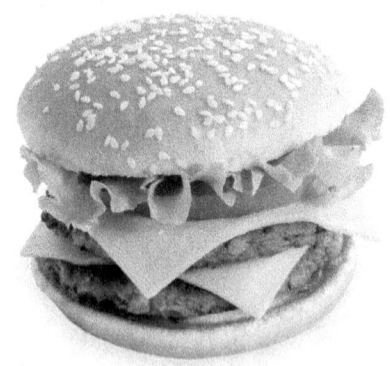

Hungry Jack's

Category	Item	% Sugar
Whoppers	Double Whopper	2.6 %
	Double Whopper Cheese	2.7 %
	Ultimate Double Whopper	2.6 %
Beef	Bacon Deluxe	2.2 %
	Hashbrown Cheeseburger	2.4 %
Chicken	Grilled Chicken Classic	2.8 %
	Grilled Chicken Peri Peri	3.0 %
	Grilled Chicken Cheesy Bacon	2.7 %
	Grilled Chicken Cheesy Bacon Peri Peri	2.8 %
	Chicken Royale	2.9 %
	Tendercrisp Classic	2.5 %
	Tendercrisp Peri Peri	2.5 %
	Chicken Crunch Classic	2.0 %
	Chicken Crunch Peri Peri	2.1 %
	Chicken Nuggets 12 Pack	0.5 %
Premium	Tendercrisp Cheesy Bacon	2.4 %
	Tendercrisp Cheesy Bacon Peri Peri	2.5 %
Sides	Onion Rings	1.9 %
	Fries	0.5 %
Breakfast	Sausage & Egg Muffin	1.6 %
	Bacon & Egg Muffin	1.9 %
	Sausage & Egg Muffin Omelette	2.4 %
	Bacon & Egg Muffin Omelette	2.9 %
	Hash Brown	0.9 %

Pizza Hut

Note: These figures have not been adjusted for lactose (in the cheese) content as it is difficult to accurately estimate. All figures would be lower when adjusted for lactose.

Category	Item	% Sugar
Classics	Loaded Ham	2.2 %
	Big Cheese	2.3 %
	Margheritaville	2.5 %
Loaded Classics	Loaded Pepperoni	1.8 %
	Veggie Trio	2.7 %
	Garlic Chook	2.8 %
	Mediterranean	1.7 %
Favourites	Super Supreme	2.7 %
	New Yorker	2.6 %
	Roast & Rasher	2.8 %
	Ultimate El Scorcho	2.8 %
Pasta	Carbonara	1.3 %
	Lasagne	1.6 %
Extras	Garlic Bread	2.7 %
	Cheesy Garlic Bread	2.7 %
	Cheesy Potato Bites	0.7 %
Chicken	Chicken Wings	0.5 %
	Fried Chicken Wings	0.6 %
Dips & Sauces	Creamy Garlic Dip	1.6 %

Domino's Pizza

Note: These figures have not been adjusted for lactose (in the cheese) content as it is difficult to accurately estimate. All figures would be lower when adjusted for lactose.

None of the pizza's currently sold by Domino's in Australia have less than 3% sugar. Some of the items on their sides menu do however still qualify.

Category	Item	% Sugar
Bread Sides	Chips	0.2 %
	Garlic Bread	2.9 %
Chicken Sides	Mild Kickers	0.4 %
	Spicy Kickers	0.4 %
	Chipotle Kickers	1.1 %
	Ribs	1.0 %
	Spicy Wings	0.8 %
	Oven Roast Wings	0.5 %
	Spicy Chicken Kicker Bites	1.4 %
Dipping Sauces	Garlic Mayo	3.0 %

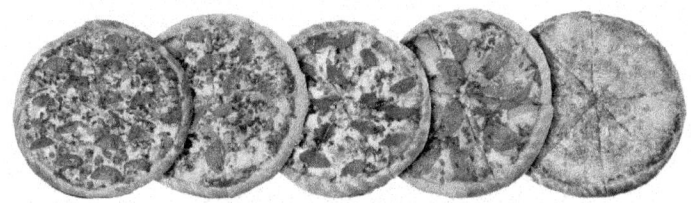

KFC

Category	Item	% Sugar
Twisters	BLT Twister	2.1%
	Regular Twister	2.1%
	Mex Fresh Twister	2.5%
Chicken	Popcorn Chicken	0.5%
	Original Recipe Chicken	1.0%
	Wicked Wings	1.6%
	SoSalad & Crispy Strips	2.4%
	SoSalad & Grilled Chicken Strips	2.4%
Snacks	Crispy Strip Snackbox	0.5%
	Grilled Taster Box	0.5%
	Nuggets Snackbox	0.5%
	Popcorn Chicken Snackbox	0.5%
	Wicked Wings Snackbox	1.0%
	BLT Snack Twister	2.0%
Extras	Gravy	0.1%
	Potato & Gravy	0.1%
	Seasoned Chips	0.5%
Breakfast	Hash Brown	0.5%

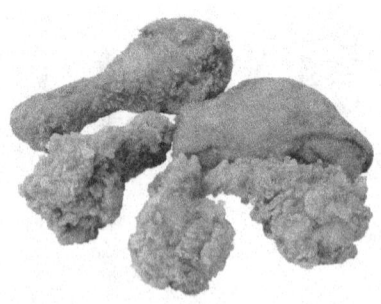

Red Rooster

Category	Item	% Sugar
Roast Chicken	Whole Roast Chicken	0.4 %
	Classic Chicken Salad	1.8 %
	Spicy Chicken Salad	2.1 %
	Classic Roast	1.7 %
	Wholesome Roast	2.3 %
Burgers, Rolls & Wraps	Caesar Roast Chicken Roll	2.2 %
	Roast Chicken & Gravy Roll	2.7 %
	Salad Roast Chicken Roll	3.0 %
	Flayva Wrap	0.4 %
	Caesar Wrap	1.8 %
	Classic Rippa	2.3 %
	Original Crispy Burger	2.7 %
Stacked Packs	Fully Loaded Packs	0.8 %
	Tropicana Pack	1.8 %
	Power Pack	0.1 %
	Legends Pack	0.8 %
Flathead Fish	Fish & Chips	0.6 %
	Fish Wrap	1.0 %
	Fish & Chips Feast	0.6 %

More Information

Still haven't found what you're looking for? I also maintain a database of over 2,000 foods including restaurant meals typically found in Asian and Mediterranean restaurants.

You can search the database for free at www.davidgillespie.org

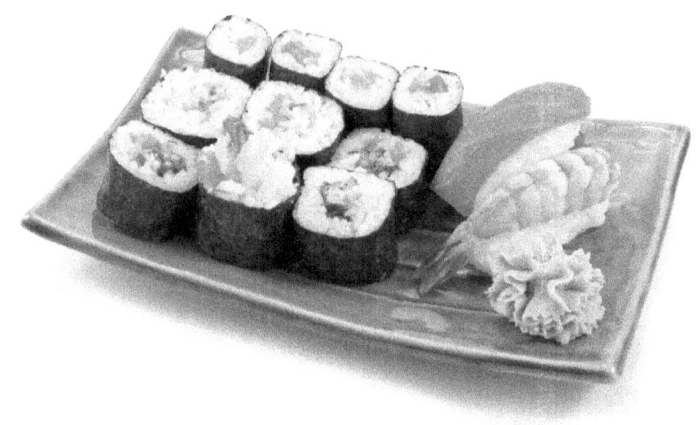

Published by the Morton Gillespie Pty Ltd
PO Box 196, Cannon Hill QLD 4170 Australia

davidgillespie.org

ISBN 978-0-9874577-5-2

Design and layout: Charlotte Gelin Design
Photographs: iStock

www.ingramcontent.com/pod-product-compliance
Lightning Source LLC
Chambersburg PA
CBHW072201280526
45788CB00002B/822